B. Luban-Plozza W. Pöldinger F. Kröger

Psychosomatic Disorders in General Practice

Third, Revised and Enlarged Edition

Translated and Revised from the German by G. Blythe

Foreword by M. Balint

With 18 Figures and 18 Tables

Springer-Verlag
Berlin Heidelberg New York London Paris
Tokyo Hong Kong Barcelona Budapest

Prof. Dr. Dr. hc. Boris Luban-Plozza
Clinica Santa Croce, Psychosomatic Department
6600 Locarno, Switzerland

Prof. Dr. Walter Pöldinger
Psychiatrische Universitätsklinik
Wilhelm-Klein-Straße 27, 4025 Basel, Switzerland

Dr. Friedebert Kröger
Rheinisch-Westfälische Technische Hochschule Aachen
Klinik für Psychosomatische Medizin
W-5100 Aachen, Bundesrepublik Deutschland

Translator:
George Blythe, Spechtstraße 3, 4106 Therwil, Switzerland

Previous editions published by © Editiones Roche, F. Hoffmann-La Roche Ltd, Basle, Switzerland

---

ISBN-13: 978-3-540-54556-9 e-ISBN-13: 978-3-642-76940-5
DOI: 10.1007/978-3-642-76940-5

Library of Congress Cataloging-in-Publication Data. Luban-Plozza, Boris. [Psychosomatisch Kranke in der Praxis. English] Psychosomatic disorders in general practice / B. Luban-Plozza, W. Pöldinger, F. Kröger. — 3rd, rev., and enl. ed. p. cm. Translation of: Der psychosomatisch Kranke in der Praxis. Includes bibliographical references and index.
ISBN-13: 978-3-540-54556-9
1. Medicine, Psychosomatic. I. Pöldinger, W. (Walter) II. Kröger, F. (Friedebert) III. Title.
RC49.L8213 1991. 616.08 — dc20.

Typesetting: Best-set Typesetter Ltd., Hong Kong
19/3130-543210 – Printed on acid-free paper

Foreword to the First Edition

This book is addressed first and foremost to the neophyte, that is to the doctor who, although properly educated in the traditional 'illness-centred medicine' is ill at ease in face of the many patients whose case histories cannot be understood and whose complaints cannot be helped on the basis of what he has learned.

Here, then, new ways of thinking and of acting are offered to him, not by devaluating his present knowledge and skills, but by using them as a basis upon which to extend his therapeutic resources.

As the first step the authors demonstrate that, in addition to the traditional understanding of the signs and symptoms of illness in terms of pathophysiological changes of the body and its functions, various diseases can also be understood as the expression of the patient's affective state, his unresolved personality conflicts and his difficulties in social adaptation. They then demonstrate the usefulness of this way of thinking. They discuss in detail the fundamental difference between the traditional way of 'taking a medical history' which, in fact, is hardly more than getting the patient to answer the items of a complicated questionnaire, and the new way of 'listening' which encourages the patient to tell his doctor not only the detailed history of his illness but also all his realistic and unrealistic fantasies and fears which are either provoked by, or expressed through, his illness. It is duly emphasized that this new way amounts to an 'examination by the patient himself' in which process the doctor's task is to help the patient to a better understanding of himself by acting as a mirror.

The danger that the doctor attaches too much significance to a possibly unimportant 'organic' symptom during the diagnostic period is properly emphasized. This usually leads to a situation in which all the patient's complaints are seen in terms of this symptom. Once a 'name' has been given to the patient's frightening fantasies and disquieting sensations it is most difficult to dislodge.

The authors take a critical view of the habitual procedure in psychosomatic conditions: as a first step the doctor undertakes a physical examination; when he is convinced that no organic abnormalities can be found, he 'reassures' the patient that he is completely healthy; all of us know how questionable the results of this reassurance are.

If the doctor knows the patient fairly well, he might try to 'advise' him how to live, how to behave. Such advice is always well meant but its therapeutic efficiency is rather doubtful.

In addition, if he feels that still more is needed, the doctor writes a prescription according to the symptomatology presented: an antidepressant for tiredness and exhaustion, sadness and despair, or a tranquilizer for complaints such as anxiety or excitation. The authors raise the justified question, is this procedure correct? And if it is, under what conditions and in what indications should these drugs be given? This of course is not an easy question to answer, all the more so since the answer depends as much on the doctor's personality and convictions as on the patient's complaints.

The authors therefore propose the principle that psychotherapy should never replace the traditional medical treatment, only complement it. Unquestionably this principle is safe and sensible, but one may ask whether it is always therapeutically efficient.

In this book Luban-Plozza and Pöldinger make a serious attempt to elucidate these complicated questions from as many angles as possible. In addition to discussing the influence of the doctor's therapeutic approach on the development of the psychosomatic complaint they also stress the repercussions of the changed atmosphere created by the Health Services in various countries. An attempt is made to discover whether the patient's personal responsibility for his illness and recovery is diminished, and whether it can be replaced by impersonal insurance or state systems. This process is further reinforced by the development of the various social services all over the Western world which try to take away still more of the patient's personal responsibility, almost saying 'If you are so weak, here we are to help you, lean on us'. The difficulties that this changed atmosphere puts in the way of the proper treatment of psychosomatic conditions are discussed.

This book will serve as a useful guide to any doctor who wishes to know more about this complex field of medicine.

MICHAEL BALINT †, LONDON
(1896–1970)

Preface to the Third Edition

Closely geared to general practice yet without neglecting basic theory, this book has retained so much appeal among readers as to warrant a third edition. We assume that the work has retained its place among the leading publications on psychosomatics because it embodies our strong interest in the 'here and now' of medical practice.

The timing of this thoroughly revised and enlarged edition appears opportune as psychosomatic basic care and the medicine of dialogue acquire more meaning in daily routine practice, and as the need for basic information increases.

We conceive psychosomatics to be an integral part of medicine. When we speak of 'psychosomatic disorders' in this book, our premise is that somatic and psychosocial aspects play an important role in their pathogenesis and course. This notion constitutes the very basis of what is understood as psychosomatic medical treatment. Such a point of departure calls for a consistent spirit of cooperation with regard to the problems involved. This alone satisfies the initial requirement of simultaneously considering both the somatic and psychosocial aspects of health and illness.

Understanding and action are impossible without resort to some form of theoretical framework. The German neurologist Victor von Weizsäcker founded the notion that psychosomatic medicine had to be depth psychological or nothing. The development of psychoanalytic theory thus is at the base of psychosomatic practice, which however is being extended by modern ideas to improve our understanding of symptoms, as for example in general-systems theory, by the stress concept, and by basic biological and social psychiatric aspects. We prefer an approach orientated towards patients and problems to one deriving exclusively from one specific, theoretical line of thought.

We the authors are closely associated and have, in this as in other editions, had a complementary effect on broadening one another's knowledge and experience. Moreover, F. Kröger, a member of the younger generation, is a coauthor of this edition, further broadening our experience.

As was the case with previous editions, this book is suited to the needs of all physicians in private practice, clinicians, and other hospital staff. It has also been our intent to make the book attractive to medical students and to open up fresh vistas on psychosomatics, not only to all those working in the various fields of health care but also to the interested layman. An attempt has been made to retain spontaneity and frankness of dialogue when comparing the various opinions and schools of thought.

We are particularly grateful to the following specialists who worked with us on this publication: Professor M. Berger (gynecological disorders), Drs. M. Fisch and E. Streich-Schlossmacher (psychological and psychosomatic aspects of dentistry), Dr. R. Hohmeister (musculoskeletal disorders), and Professor A. Krebs (skin diseases).

Locarno/Basle/Heidelberg 1991

Boris Luban-Plozza
Walter Pöldinger
Friedebert Kröger

Contents

1 Psychosomatic Groundwork

1.1 Historical Introduction

Research has shown that successful practical medicine has, from its very inception, always been psychosomatic in its essence. In this vein, the American psychiatrist O.S. English described 'psychosomatic' as being a relatively new term for one of the rudiments of medicine that is as old as the art itself.

The idea that it is impossible to separate the health of the body from that of the mind was put forward in such early works as the Book of Job.

Plato also expressed this point of view in *Charmides:* 'The cure of many diseases is unknown to the physicians of Hellas, because they disregard the whole, which ought to be studied also, for the part can never be well unless the whole is well.'

The contrasting natures of the Hippocratic school of *Kos*, with its dynamic, humoral and psychic (hence also psychosomatic) concepts, and the school of *Knidos*, which was mechanistically and organicistically orientated, are well known.

An interesting diagnosis is that made by Erasistratos of the Alexandrian school of the third century before Christ; this man was summoned by the King of Syria to examine his son, who was suffering from what was thought to be an incurable disease. While the physician was taking the patient's pulse, the beautiful Stratonike came into the room. From the psychosomatic reaction of the heart beat, Erasistratos immediately realized that the young man's illness had been caused by his hopeless love for his father's second wife. In order that his son might be cured the father was willing to separate from his wife.

The three great philosophers of the seventeenth century also concerned themselves with the body–mind problem:

Descartes (1596–1650) devised a complex theory on the interaction between the corporeal world (*extensio*) and consciousness or soul (*cogitatio*). He counts as one of the most prominent exponents of body mind dualism.

In his work on anthropology, Spinoza (1632–1677) put forward the thesis that all events in the body had their parallels in the mind, which was nothing more than the idea of the real body (ideoplasia).

Leibniz (1646–1716) replaced psychophysical interaction by pre-established harmony: a predetermined accord exists between each of the events taking place in the body and in the mind.

The originator of the term 'psychosomatic' is held to be the German practitioner Johann Christian Heinroth (1773–1843), who later became Professor of Psychiatry at Leipzig University. In 1818, Heinroth declared: 'Insomnia is usually psychic and somatic in origin but any phase of life can itself constitute the sole cause of the disorder.' In 1822, Jacobi introduced the term 'somato-psychic' in order to stress the predominance of somatic factors in the development of certain disorders.

Groos also adopted a psychosomatic standpoint when he wrote in 1824: 'If we seek the first cause of the most diverse illnesses, we can find it in the directly injurious effect of the passions on the body.' He worked on the assumption that 'the essence of mental illness is of psychosomatic nature' and took what he believed to be a conciliatory position in the old controversy between the psychicists and the somaticists.

A classic piece of self-observation was made by the French clinician Trousseau in 1830, who described his experience as follows: 'The worst attack of asthma that I have ever suffered occurred under the following circumstances: I suspected that my coachman was stealing oats from me, and in order to clarify matters I went to the barn and had the stocks of oats measured. While this was being done I suffered an extremely severe attack of asthma which was obviously brought on by the emotional feelings aroused by the thought of the minor domestic theft.'

A very modern view was expressed by Maudsley as early as 1876: 'If the emotion be not discharged in outward bodily activity or in suitable mental action, it will act upon the internal viscera and derange their functions; sorrow is soon discharged by passionate wailing and weeping . . .'

However, the terms 'psychosomatic disorders' and 'psychosomatic medicine' have only found general acceptance in the last few decades, after the adjective 'psychosomatic' was again brought into use in 1922 by the Viennese psychoanalyst Felix Deutsch. He described psychosomatic medicine as 'applied psychoanalysis in medicine'.

Although other psychoanalysts such as Groddeck (1961), Ferenczi (1965), and Jelliffe (after Alexander 1948) had turned their attention to somatic disorders some ten years before, they described them as organ neuroses and organ psychoses (Meng 1934, 1935).

It was particularly Groddeck who attempted in the course of his lively and brilliant discussions with Freud to outline how organic diseases ultimately have a psychological nature. He took the stand that disease was somehow linked with the id (or *Es* – a term he himself coined), with the 'force that leads our lives, while we think we are leading them'.

Von Krehl, von Weizsäcker and von Bergmann should be counted among the pioneers of psychosomatic medicine who stemmed from the field of internal medicine.

Deutsch (1939) later emigrated to the United States where he became the progenitor of an American psychosomatic medicine that in its early stages was predominantly psychoanalytically orientated. Among its other pioneers were Dunbar (1947, 1948) and Alexander (1939, 1948).

Judging from the number of publications, interest in psychosomatic medicine has since increased tremendously. As early as 1954, Dunbar listed no fewer than 5,000 publications from this field in her book *Emotions and Bodily Changes*.

This number has now more than doubled, and the authors are no longer drawn mainly from the ranks of the psychoanalysts as was still the case only a few years ago. Psychosomatic correlates are acknowledged as a clinical reality in most fields of medicine.

The Development of Psychotherapy

Whereas the term 'psychiatry' covers all theories, no matter how great the differences between those that attempt to offer a scientific explanation of mental disturbances, 'psychotherapy' is always directed towards the individual and is concerned with his particularities and his unique destiny.

It would be fitting at this juncture to mention just a few stages in the history of psychotherapy – from the magic of all ages through the Indian Yoga doctrines of 'concentration' and 'meditation' to the Western theories of systematic psychotherapy with which we are familiar today and which have their origins in 'animal magnetism'. Originally dominated by metaphysical theories and mystical beliefs, psychotherapy only gradually evolved into a scientific discipline.

The Precursors

All the modern methods involving techniques of suggestion are to some extent derived from the practices of the Viennese physician Franz Anton Mesmer (1734–1815). In its early years hypnosis was used mainly in France; Liébeault (1823–1904) founded a hospital in Nancy where he employed hypnosis in the treatment of physical disorders, suggesting to his patients that their symptoms had disappeared.

The necessity for a rigorous scientific approach to techniques of suggestion was recognized at a very early stage. Research into the effects of suggestion, under hypnosis or otherwise, drew attention to the fact that the same results could be obtained by autosuggestion without the constant intervention of the suggestor. The pharmacist Coué from Nancy was an enthusiastic champion of the efficacy of this procedure.

In Berne Dubois (1848–1918), who was first and foremost a practising physician and not a psychiatrist, maintained that he was able to reassure his patients simply by talking to them (persuasion technique). He attempted to show them that their hypochondriacal ideas, which constituted the focal point of their mental disorders, were unfounded. However, appeals to reason cannot eliminate the true causes of disease, since psychogenic disorders do not arise from faulty thought processes but have much deeper origins. In order to discern and treat the latter, Sigmund Freud (1856–1939) developed psychoanalysis.

The Decisive Turning Point

Freud began his career in Vienna, devoting his attention first to the study of the central nervous system. In 1885, he went to the Salpêtrière, where Charcot, with the aid of hypnosis, was able to elicit and eliminate symptoms in hysterical subjects more or less at will. This was the first application of a psychotherapeutic technique, although it was used more for research than for treatment. But the hypnosis relied on the principle of authority: the curative effects disappeared if authority was lost.

Freud later went to Nancy where he joined Liébeault and his assistant Bernheim (1873–1939) who were using hypnosis for therapeutic purposes. Once returned to Vienna, he was stimulated by the views of Breuer and developed a wealth of new ideas.

In Vienna Breuer, a colleague of the physiologist Ibering, had discovered the cathartic method which influenced Freud. It was with Breuer that Freud made his first psychoanalytical observations, the subject being a girl who was cured of severe hysteria; this patient was induced, under hypnosis, to recall experiences she had previously been unable to admit (*Studien über Hysterie,* 1895). However, Freud soon realized that hypnosis did not have a favourable effect on the treatment process and that events could be recalled without it. Hypnosis was therefore abandoned and replaced by the technique of free association. It is easy to imagine the effect this technique had at a time when there was so much that was 'not talked about'.

The abandonment of hypnosis in psychotherapy paved the way for further methodological developments and true psychoanalysis. Freud discovered that repressed experiences relegated to the unconscious exerted, by way of the preconscious, a considerable 'dynamic' effect on the whole personality. Events which were no longer part of the conscious mind exerted a marked influence from the other side of the threshold of consciousness. These discoveries led to the theory of the unconscious which, while inaccessible as such to the subject, can be rendered conscious by means of analysis. Experiences which cannot be handled in the conscious or the preconscious are repressed by defence mechanisms into the unconscious (displacement). As we shall see, the emotional factors involved in psychosomatic disorders are of an unconscious (and neurotic) nature.

In the very early stages of psychoanalysis the all-important discovery was made that dreams provided a means of reaching the unconscious. In addition to dreams and free association, the latter being fostered in a relaxed mental state such as is aimed at in psychoanalysis, symptomatic acts (slips of the tongue, mistakes in writing, lapses of memory, mislaying an object) also give important clues to unconscious processes.

Alongside the discovery of resistance and defence mechanisms and the realization that the unconscious could be reached through dreams, free association and symptomatic acts, another methodologically and therapeutically important phenomenon also came to light, namely transference. Every patient receiving psychoanalytical treatment to a greater or lesser extent transfers his feelings to the analyst, displacing his memories of the most important people in his childhood (father, mother, and possibly siblings).

The phenomena of transference and resistance, together with the Oedipus complex and infantile sexuality, are among the key factors in psychoanalysis. As Freud said: 'The assumption of unconscious mental processes, the recognition of the theory of resistance and repression, and the appreciation of sexuality and the Oedipus complex constitute the main elements of psychoanalysis and the basic premises of its theory; no one should consider himself a psychoanalyst if he cannot sanction them' (Freud 1916/1961b).

The psychic 'energy' of repressed experience and the dynamics of the 'mechanism' of symptom formation in hysterical and other neurotic syndromes stem far more from a driving force in the individual than from conflict between the conscious and the unconscious. Freud called this force 'libido', by which he understood the energy of the sexual drive. This drive, which serves both to preserve the species and to satisfy the pleasure principle, is particularly likely to come into conflict with prevailing moral laws. Even if it is repressed it retains its original energy and may take the form of symptoms (conversion symptoms). It can lead to diffuse anxiety (anxiety neurosis) or become attached to inappropriate objects, which undergo secondary eroticization. At best, insufficient release of libido will result in sublimation, the originally sexual libido being converted into intellectual or artistic activity.

The importance of the sex drive, which Freud only later contrasted with the destructive tendency, the death instinct, was given open expression for the first time by psychoanalysis.

Freud's sexual theory differentiates between the predominant component instinct and the object relationship determined by this instinct. A further differentiation is made between the various sexual phases in human development. Freud attributed the pleasure derived by the infant when feeding at his mother's breast to the oral phase of sexuality. The anal phase is the stage when the child learns cleanliness; the infant's excretory function is experienced as pleasurable and the parents' attempts at training as 'frustrating', i.e. prohibitory and unpleasurable. This is followed by the genital phase – a term which led to a great deal of misunderstanding. Later psychoanalytical research showed that the child's experiences during these three phases were crucial to his later development. The phases themselves, which are interrupted by the latency period, may in fact persist to some extent or become 'socialized'. In extreme situations a person may regress to one of these phases.

Psychoanalysis represents an attempt to examine the human personality in depth, going beyond the investigation of the content of consciousness. The tripartite division of the personality into the id, the ego and the superego was later adopted by many schools of psychology, although different terms were employed.

The id is the realm of the unconscious, of the instincts and the vital forces; it supports and influences the other two realms. The ego, which becomes crystallized during the rebellious phase, is responsible for conscious parts of the personality, self-awareness and voluntary behaviour; the ego is the organized part of the personality whereas the id is 'unorganized'. The superego conforms to the obligating – restrictive but guiding – rules of society and is therefore responsible for conscience and morality. Using the above terminology, the aim of analytical treatment as Freud saw it – an aim which he himself described as utopian – was that 'the ego should take over from the id', i.e. that the unconscious thought processes should as far as possible be uncovered and rendered conscious so that they could be integrated into the existing organization.

Actual conflict, triggered off by 'temptation and failure situations', is intensified by the residuum of unresolved childhood experiences. The consciousness may finally become dependent on infantile and repressed instinctual desires.

'Conflict as an experience represents a clash between at least two incompatible tendencies which act simultaneously as motives determining experience and behaviour' (Bräutigam 1969). Much can be learned from attempting to identify such tendencies. Whether conflicts of this type produce constructive-creative states of tension or gradually evolve into illness is closely bound up with the personality of the individual involved.

The psychoanalytical school also opened the way to new psychotherapeutic measures, which in part are based on one or another of the theories put forward only tentatively by Freud.

C.G. Jung (1875–1961) used the Freudian term 'libido' in the wider sense of a 'pathoenergic' principle comprising two mutually opposed forces, one centripetal (introversion) and the other centrifugal (extraversion). He is best remembered, however, for his theory of the collective unconscious which he saw as innate and permitting understanding of the universally human meaning behind even foreign cultures. Jung investigated and correlated the concepts of conscious, unconscious and instinct. From this approach grew his theory of archetypes. Archetypes, which in their symbolism may also express religious feelings, have the meaning of collective symbols.

The aim of psychotherapy as Jung understood it differed from that of Freudian psychoanalysis. Freud likened the analytical method to the surgeon's scalpel which cuts away diseased tissue and leaves Nature to heal the wound. He expressly warned against direct interference in the life of the neurotic with practical advice and moral or intellectual instructions. Jung's aim, on the other hand, was not only to remove what is diseased but also to add what is healthy and assist the neurotic to gain an advantage in mental maturity that even the 'normal' person does not possess.

Whereas Freud says that 'the ego should take over from the id', the demand Jung makes of the individuation process is that 'the self should take over from the ego'. Jung uses 'self' to refer to the whole psyche, both the spiritual, superconscious region of the unconscious and the instinctual subconscious region.

The purpose of the individuation process is to synthesize the various aspects of the conscious and the unconscious mind. Step by step the ego, in a series of 'transmutations', comes to grips with the archetypes of the collective unconscious. In Jung's words (1950), 'If man is to live he must fight and sacrifice his retrograde yearnings in order to ascend to his own heights.' In Freudian language this means that he must come to terms with reality.

Alfred Adler (1870–1937), in his 'individual psychology', interpreted neurosis as an existential crisis affecting the whole person. He saw the basic phenomenon of psychic disorders not as stemming from the drives but as the 'nervous character', i.e. the inadequate attitude to life and one's fellow men acquired during childhood and leading in some cases to a striving for power. In the mentally ill Adler saw a feeling of weakness and helplessness which he described as the 'inferiority complex'. He also postulated that certain organs were 'inferior' (locus minoris resistentiae, miopragia) and that a corresponding 'symptom choice' occurred. Adler's individual psychology regards nervous symptoms as the final expression of the struggle to overcome feelings of inadequacy. The development of 'nervous' symptoms is seen as a 'flight into illness', a 'striving for power' or a 'masculine protest' which draws attention to itself, the striving coming into conflict with the feeling for the community.

In this context we should also mention Stekel (1920, 1927) who pioneered 'surprise' therapy, a technique which involved a rapid and intuitive intervention by the doctor that enabled actual conflicts at the root of neuroses to be uncovered and dealt with.

Szondi (1968) developed a depth-psychological technique which in particular enabled unconscious ancestral desires to become conscious. In Szondi's 'fate analysis' the individual is confronted with his unconscious 'destiny possibilities' and presented with the choice of a better personal form of existence.

Maeder (1953, 1963), the clergyman Pfister (1921) and Tournier (1959, 1961, 1964) in particular attempted to explain the relationship between the problems of theology and depth psychology.

In addition to differentiating between life and death instincts, Schultz-Hencke (1970) distinguished between those of possession, recognition, tenderness and aggression. He described his approach as neopsychoanalytical and tried to break away from the rigidity of the genotype concept in psychopathy and expand it in accordance with his theory of neuroses. He always included physiological considerations in his psychoanalytical working hypotheses and outlined at a very early stage which somatic functional disorders were attributable to the repression of certain emotions, needs and impulses. Erich Fromm (1966, 1968) has also been classed among this neo-Freudian school, wrongly in his opinion. He devoted particular attention to social factors and has made important contributions towards an 'active psychotherapy' in a sociopsychoanalytical sense.

The ideas of the internist and neurologist Viktor von Weizsäcker were strongly influenced by Freudian views. He coined the phrase: 'Psychosomatic medicine must be depth psychological in essence or nothing at all.' The consistent application of psychological principles at the patient's bedside finally led him to postulate that the physician's duty is not confined to repairing the sick machinery of the body. Both doctor and patient should rather try to understand the patient's life history and the significance of the illness in the context of the severe vicissitudes in human affairs, making the patient aware of his existential crisis or its abrupt inception. Essential to his anthropological way of thought is that the *patient be included* in the medical concept.

Following on from Kierkegaard, Heidegger (1963) singled out anxiety and death as the fundamental conditions of human existence. His writings attempt to discover deep meaning in the very words of the language. He thus interprets 'existence' (*Dasein*) as meaning 'being-in-the-world' while the man 'waits outside with things and people'. This science makes use of phenomenological methods of investigation; it strives to clarify the phenomena of existence with the greatest possible attention to subtleties of detail.

Existential analysis was introduced into psychiatry by Binswanger (1955) for the study of affective and mental disorders and by Boss (1954) as the starting point for important psychosomatic studies and psychotherapeutic training.

In contrast with the exponents of psychoanalysis and existential analysis, Staehelin (1969) believes that human nature involves more than the first reality of man's individual biographical and conditional finiteness and mortality. He describes a second reality peculiar to man which is characterized by spatial and spiritual infinite and immortal qualities, a reality which belongs to the realm of ultimate unconditionality, the realm of the absolute. The fundamental confidence of the healthy man is rooted in this second reality. This type of 'reality analysis' might also be of value to complement psychotherapy.

Jores (1970), a specialist in internal medicine, identifies as specifically 'human disorders' a group of disorders in which not so much physical damage but rather the patient's problems with life and his human failings are expressed. They do not occur in animals unless their psychosocial environment is first changed. This was difficult to understand since the organs that undergo structural or functional changes in the disorders concerned are to a large extent anatomically similar in humans and animals and their physiology is also approximately the same. From this Jores concluded that if the difference were not biological then it must lie in human characteristics. In his view only psychotherapy is able to call a halt to a pathological process of this type, by altering, in the course of the discussions, the patient's faulty 'outlook on life', which is at the root of his 'specifically human' disorder.

1.2 Psychosomatic Correlates

What is the reason for this new interest on the part of the general practitioner?

In the last few decades it has become increasingly clear that the usual distinction drawn between 'organic' and 'functional' disorders is questionable.

Doctors have begun to realize that disorders often occur against a background of many factors. Out of this there has also grown an interest in the role of psychological and social factors in illness, and as a result of this new orientation medical practice has come to be regarded in a broader context. The patient is no longer merely the bearer of a diseased organ; he is thought of as a whole person and treated accordingly. The aim of psychosomatic medicine accords well with this new conception even though, strictly speaking, it concentrates mainly on disorders whose etiology and pathogenesis are dominated by emotional factors.

Modern medicine must be understood and practised in the light of the psychosomatic factors involved if therapy is not to run the risk of becoming a sterile 'prosthetic' technique. In other words, *psychological understanding,* the desire to penetrate to the patient's intimate emotional problems, should be just as much a part of the doctor's equipment as any drug or instrument – all the more so since statistics and conservative estimates show that about a third of the patients who visit their general practitioner are suffering from functional or emotionally induced disorders. Inner conflicts, neurotic mechanisms and psychoreactive factors influence the course, duration and character of organic disorders and possibly even resistance to therapy.

Many authors see psychosomatic medicine as a healthy reaction to the depersonalized medicine which has arisen as a result of extreme specialization (a necessary evil) and which, with its increasingly heavy reliance on technical aids to diagnosis and treatment, has wrought fundamental changes in the doctor-patient relationship. Added to this we have the structuring of diseases to be outnumbered by chronic disorders with all the social problems they involve.

From what has been said it will be clear that the psychosomatic approach calls for a fundamental change in medical attitudes. It will represent a genuine advance provided it does not overshadow the knowledge so far gained from studies in anatomy, biochemistry and pathophysiology. The aim should rather be to complement the achievements of these disciplines from both the therapeutic and the diagnostic points of view.

Of particular relevance in this connection are the comments of Hoff and Ringel (1964): '. . . one should never attempt to explain the pathogenesis of any disorder on the basis of psychological factors alone. The few attempts that have been made at this have been much to the detriment of our subject since such one-sided attitudes serve only to reinforce the resistance that already exists in many medical circles to psychosomatic thinking. Thus, we cannot lay too much stress on the fact that psychogenic factors represent only one aspect of pathology; they must be taken in conjunction with other aspects before we can arrive at the *comprehensive approach* which is nowadays becoming so important in the field of pathogenesis.'

It must be remembered that psychosomatic medicine is not, as is often maintained, concerned with purely theoretical speculations; it is based on the fact that emotions can cause marked changes in organ function – something which has time and again been demonstrated and confirmed experimentally (Alexander et al. 1968; Hahn 1979; Uexküll 1979; Weiner et al. 1957).

The following section will deal with various concepts of psychophysiological connections. The linchpins and focuses of such concepts are to be found partly in physiological observations and partly in the psychoanalytical approach.

1.2.1 Psychophysiological Connections

The Conditioned Reflex

The Russian physiologist Ivan Pavlov (1849–1936) differentiated between two types of nerve functions: those of the lower nervous system located in the spinal cord and certain parts of the brain mainly served the purpose of integrating relationships between different parts of the body, while higher nerve functions were said to involve the cerebral hemispheres and adjoining subcortex and guarantee the normal, complex relationships existing between the entire organism and its environment (Pavlov).

He made a further differentiation in the higher nerve functions between conditioned and unconditioned reflexes. According to Pavlov, the inborn, subcortical unconditioned reflexes served to fulfil such elementary needs as searching for food. They correspond to what is generally understood by instincts and drives. Conditioned reflexes, however, are not inborn but acquired. Pavlov described them as 'elementary, objective thinking' which enables the organism to adapt to the external world.

Unlike the events giving rise to unconditioned reflexes, the stimulus triggering off conditioned reflexes passes through no genetically predetermined pathways; such an acquired reflex is dependent on the formation of new functional connections in the nervous system by repetitive stimuli. This can be achieved in animals experimentally by pairing an unconditioned stimulus with an originally unconditioned reflex, e.g. repeatedly offering food while a bell is rung simultaneously. After a time, the ringing of the bell alone will elicit salivation. The conditioned reflex has thus replaced the original stimulus by dint of the learning process or conditioning. The resulting response, now a conditioned reflex, does not undergo any basic alteration. In man, language constitutes a further signal system for establishing such connections.

The model provided by conditioned reflexes is of interest in formulating psychosomatic theories in that asthmatic attacks could be produced experimentally in guinea pigs with antigen or histamine and, after merely five reinforcements of an acoustic signal, the attacks were precipitated by the signal alone (Petzold, Reindell 1977). It was also possible to produce 'experimental neurosis' in animals. If two conditioned reflexes with opposing reactions are created and the triggering stimuli applied simultaneously, the animals develop behavioural disturbances and autonomic disorders to the point of causing irreversible organic lesions (hypertension and myocardial infarction).

Pavlov himself indicated the limited possibilities of extrapolating such experimental findings, particularly those obtained from laboratory animals, to humans. On account of difficulties in methodology, he chose to disregard the inner world of subjective and imaginative experience of the living organisms on which he experimented and remain strictly in the role of a physiologist, even regarding emotional conflicts. In other words, he restricted himself to making objective observations concerned exclusively with 'external phenomena and their relationships'.

The physiologist Schäfer writes: 'Our impression is that certain situations trigger off certain emotions. These emotions are capable of both increasing gastric secretion and inhibiting the production of protective colloids and may thus ultimately result in ulcer formation. The scientific problems present difficulties because we are correlating a somatic disorder with a situation that triggers off emotions. The presenting disorder can be described fairly well; the specialist can easily detect a stomach ulcer. It is very much more difficult to define a situation. Furthermore, the causative factor is not the situation itself but the way in which the individual reacts to it. This, for example, is the reason why Christian et al. (1966) stress the importance of personalities at risk. Such correlations are only feasible if large numbers of people are investigated, and even then a degree of uncertainty remains in the assessment of individual cases.

'A statistical evaluation of such psychosomatic interrelationships can be performed by making a detailed analysis of case observations (case team work) and then attempting to evolve a rational theory of the disorder; to this end, additional physiological experiments may be carried out on animals subjected to extreme conditions (cf. Pavlov and his followers), or serial investigations may be performed in humans (epidemiology). The animal experiments are based on the assumption that these effects are emotional and reactive in origin, i.e. that they can in some way be 'understood'. Within the framework of such a theory what happens in animals is ultimately interpreted by analogy with humans. We realize that a given situation must be a conflict situation for animals. The notion of conflict, however, derives not from animal physiology but manifestly from the world of man' (Schäfer 1968).

Despite these methodological difficulties, the school of Pavlov and certain aspects of ethology provided valuable stimuli for subsequent concepts on learning theory and behavioural therapy.

Emergency Responses

The physiologist Cannon (1871–1945) discovered in 1934 that *emergency states* predisposed the body to fight or flight. 'The physical changes that accompany certain emotions are a means to an end, they prepare the body to fight or flee. Thus rage, for example, brings with it an adjustment of the autonomic functions to external activity demands. The emotion prepares the body to cope at lightning speed with any emergencies that may arise. It is, so to speak, the mobilization order that brings to the ready the means to fight or flee.'

The following observation illustrates how deeply mere emotional involvement can effect the body functions. Cannon found that the urine of five reserves at a football match, like that of most of their team mates actually participating in the game, contained sugar even though they had not been active on the field. Furthermore, the excited spectators were also found to have sugar in their urine. Tests conducted on examination candidates also revealed the presence of sugar in the urine as an expression of anxiety.

According to Cannon man is constantly in a certain state of readiness for events that may appear as emergencies. When they occur, this preparedness is converted into adaptive physiological changes. Whether or not such events have been misinterpreted is without significance for the accompanying bodily response.

Neurophysiologists contend that all stress situations lead to an activation of the hypothalamus, which immediately sets protective and defence mechanisms in train along motor, visceral and neurohormonal pathways. At the same time signals are transmitted to the cerebral cortex so that emotion is perceived and recognized. If the threat to the organism continues, the forces maintaining the internal equilibrium must remain active longer. This can lead to peripheral functional or even organic disturbances in the systems affected.

In summary, it may be said that certain emotions trigger off certain autonomic alterations. Such an association can be described as a *psychosomatic model*. In the notion of emergency response, Cannon (1975) linked emotional experience with accompanying reactions in the body; and by introducing the emotions into this field of study, his ideas differ from those involved in the reflex model.

Stress

Selye (1946, 1959) described a *stress pathogenesis* which was an expansion of Cannon's theories and his own general *adaptation syndrome*. Under the term 'stressor' he included all the physical, chemical and emotional stress factors that act on the organism. Physical and emotional stress places a demand on the organism to adapt to the unaccustomed stressors. This is where the adaptation syndrome comes into play, a nonspecific reaction comprising three phases:

1. Stage of alarm reaction.
2. Stage of resistance.
3. Stage of exhaustion.

Selye's (1946) hypotheses were supported by animal experiments, and he was able to demonstrate humoral and morphological alterations, particularly in the adrenal medulla, in all of the above stages. The course taken by the general adaptation syndrome varies, depending on the initial conditon of the organism. While the actual adaptation of the organism takes place during the stage of resistance, this process becomes exhausted in the ensuing phase. This is followed by a collapse of the regulating mechanisms accompanied by irreversible somatic alterations.

Stress research initially revolved around studies on the effect of extreme stress situations, which place exceptional strain on the adaptational capacity of all people. Examples included confinement in concentration camps and permanent separation of infants from their mothers. Large scale studies also showed that changes in life patterns can certainly increase susceptibility to illness. The life-event research conducted by Holmes and Rahe (quoted in Blomke 1976) showed that the frequency and intensity of such changes – and thus the demand on adaptational capacity – increased before the outbreak of illness.

Engel and Schmale (1968) investigated primarily the stress reaction to real or imaginary object loss. They established that psychosomatic illness frequently occurred when the loss gave rise to feelings of helplessness and hopelessness (giving up–given up). The midpoint of stress research soon shifted to the subjective experience of external stressors. People experience demands on performance differently, in accordance with the degree of confidence they have in their own capacity, the pleasure they take in their work, and the ambitions they cherish. The mastering of a situation is determined by its individual significance.

The stress model has proved a useful bridge between physiology on the one hand and psychology and psychoanalysis on the other, as well as providing stimuli for research in psychosomatic medicine. Von Uexküll (1979) gives a comprehensive outline of the individual findings and theories offered by this model.

The term 'stress' has been adopted in a non-technical sense by the lay public and frequently used for events and demanding situations considered as onerous or worrisome. In one of his later publications, however, Selye (1975) emphasizes the need for 'stress' in every form of physical and emotional activity.

Petzold (1976) points out that despite the vagueness surrounding the term, its use has contributed to the relief of patients often subject to strong internal and external pressures, all the more so when it was increasingly difficult to find a somatic cause for their illness. 'For these patients, the term "stress" is mostly a relief, a possibility of retreating to a line from which they have a chance of building up anew', wrote Petzold, and went on to say: 'If anything at all can help psychotherapeutically, it is the verbalization of that for which the patient has no word. If the term "stress" did not exist, it would have to be invented for therapeutic reasons.'

1.2.2 Psychodynamic Concepts

Conflicts Specific to Illness – Conversion

The physician and psychoanalyst Franz Alexander (1891–1964) submitted an extensive and self-contained theory for explaining psychosomatic correlates. By a psychosomatic approach he understood the synchronous use of physiological and psychological methods and notions. His basic premise was that psychosomatic examinations require just as detailed and precise a description of psychological sequences as they do of observations made on the accompanying physiological processes. He considered that a 'constitutional X factor' must be assumed in the development of a psychosomatic disorder (Alexander 1951).

Following Freud's differentiation between conversion reactions (e.g. a hysterical gait disorder) and vegetative symptoms accompanying actual neuroses (e.g. cardiac neurosis), Alexander made a distinction between the hysterical-conversion reaction and adaptive changes in vegetative functions elicited by emotional tensions. Like Freud, he sees in the conversion reaction the symbolic expression of an emotion that could be verbalized but is repudiated and repressed owing to feelings of guilt or shame. The body then serves as the instrument of this expression.

According to Alexander, the symptoms of vegetative neurosis do not represent an attempt to express a repressed emotion but are rather concomitant physiological symptoms of certain emotional states. In this respect he tended to follow Cannon's ideas by stating: 'The elevation of blood pressure in rage, for example, does not discharge the emotional tension but is a physiological component of the complete picture of events. Rage . . . increased secretion of the gastric juices under the influence of instinctive craving for food (is) not an expression or discharge of such feelings; it is the adaptive preparation of the stomach for taking nourishment.' Alexander speaks of a vegetative neurosis when the accompanying physiological symptoms to emotional tensions persist owing to the absence of externally directed action able to discharge such affects. At a further stage the reversible functional symptoms lead to irreversible physical alterations.

The reason for the blockade of such overt action is seen by Alexander to lie in conflictual patterns that lead to the actualization of conflicts from the preverbal era of the individual. The fact that such conflicts derive from a period of limited differentiation of the emotional structure favours – along with constitutional factors – physical conversion. According to Alexander, these conflictual patterns may often only be clarified in the course of lengthy psychoanalysis.

Unlike other psychosomaticists such as Dunbar, who attempted to correlate somatic types of reaction with consistent personality profiles, Alexander devoted particular attention to identifying circumscribed conflictual patterns for certain physiological modes of reaction. His guideline for research was that specificity must be sought in the conflict situation. His model is thus often described as the 'theory of psychodynamic conflicts specific to illness'.

An initial classification was made according to the various functions of the autonomic nervous system. Alexander distinguished between sympathetic and parasympathetic states of preparedness (*Bereitstellungen*). Those evoked by the sympathetic system are to a certain extent futile if aggressive tendencies are denied expression. 'Whenever the possibility for competitive, aggresive and hostile attitudes is deliberately inhibited, the sympathetic-adrenergic system falls into a state of continual excitation. The autonomic symptoms arise from the trammeled sympathetic stimulus, which continues because it is not discharged by the flight-fight reaction.' An example given by Alexander to illustrate this was the patient with essential hypertension.

If the wish to be helped and similar passive tendencies are denied, the result is a state of futile parasympathetic preparedness. This affects primarily the gastrointestinal tract, which Alexander showed to be particularly the case in ulcer patients.

The strict distinction made between sympathetic and parasympathetic influences has been criticized by internists, as has that drawn between illness caused by hysterical-conversion reactions and vegetative neurosis. Doubt has also been cast on the theory of *specificity* (relating specific emotional conflicts to specific organ systems). Psychosomatic research is nevertheless indebted to Alexander's early work comprising extremely careful investigations and differentiated correlations between emotional experience and physiological reactions. These efforts have had a lasting effect on the development of this field of medicine.

Desomatization – Resomatization. Two-Phase Repression

Max Schur (1897–1969), medical doctor and psychoanalyst, who was Freud's personal physician from 1928 onwards, developed a model for explaining psychosomatic illness. This was based on investigations made on skin disease and later became known under the terms 'desomatization and resomatization'.

He observed that infants react in an unconscious (primary process) manner to disturbances in homeostatic equilibrium with their physiological control mechanisms. This was attributed to their underdeveloped and insufficiently differentiated psychic and somatic structures. With progressive maturation, increased structuring of the ego permits ever more conscious (secondary process) response to danger and anxiety states.

The continued development of perceptual faculties enables the child to give increasing consideration to reality, while that of memory opens up the way to foresight. Mental reflection, as well as control over drives and emotions, then become possible. During a process of desomatization the growing individual becomes increasingly independent of autonomous means of discharge for maintaining homeostasis.

However, should the ego prove susceptible to disturbance, and unconscious neurotic conflicts be activated under stressful situations, the insecurity produced may give rise to regression. If, moreover, emotional capacities for assimilation are exceeded, somatic symptoms may arise given certain predispositions and developmental states of organs and systems. The long and painful process of maturation is then to some extent quite suddenly reversed. The ego loses its capacity for secondary process thinking, it operates with non-neutralized forms of energy and is no longer able to maintain the painstakingly acquired desomatization of its reactions. This type of regression with resomatization is described as physiological regression. The conclusion may thus be drawn that the occurrence of somatic symptoms is bound up with certain ego functions. A parallel would consequently appear to exist between the predominance of primary process thinking, the failure of the neutralizing function, and the resomatization of reactions.

Alexander Mitscherlich (1956) was prompted by these ideas to develop his concept of the *two-phase defence* mechanism or *two-phase repression*. According to Mitscherlich, the primary condition of any chronic psychosomatic illness is a grave neurosis. An unpreventable crisis sets in during the first phase of repression or other defence mechanisms accompanied by neurotic symptoms. When such *psychic* response to overcoming the conflict situation is inadequate, there is a shift during a second phase to dynamic *somatic* defence mechanisms.

This model also explains the frequently observed changes in neurotic symptoms and somatic diseases. Neurotic symptoms recede distinctly when a somatic illness develops and frequently return if it is cured.

The Differentiation of Conversion Disorders

Von Uexküll (1963) leaned heavily on Cannon's emergency theory of emotions when he discussed the 'so-called psychosomatic disorders' (*Bereitstellungskrankheiten*).[1] In such conditions there is generally a swing of emotions produced by an apparently threatening event towards a bodily state of preparedness. In this reaction, the body no longer relies on common-sense judgement as to whether the danger is real but rather on emotions and affects. This state of preparedness may become chronic if its original purpose for coping with fight or flight is not carried out. The sequel may be a permanent elevation of functional organic activity and can, for example, result in ulceration owing to protracted increased secretion of gastric juices. Repetitive rises in blood pressure of psychogenic origin can lead to increased peripheral resistance and essential hypertension owing to reactive alterations in precapillary arterioles. According to von Uexküll, illness occurs because the induced state of preparedness cannot be resolved. This may be the sequel to disturbed maturation or caused by a loss in motivation due to repression.

Conversion symptoms differ from those of the above somatoform disorders in that they have underlying motivational conflicts. Repressed material in the form of impulses, wishes and fantasies then manifests itself as 'fragmentary acts' in hysterical symptoms. These symptoms have expressive significance, and unlike those of the other somatoform disorders are seen as cryptic attempts at communication.

As with von Weizsäcker's gestalt cycle or perceptual feedback concept (1940/50), von Uexküll's model of the situational cycle anticipated present concepts of a cybernetic model and a general-systems approach to psychosomatic medicine.

---

[1] Disorders of the disposition of emotions which anticipate or prepare one for action (Weiner).

Alexithymia

The term 'alexithymia' (*a* for lack of, *lexis* for word and *thymos* for emotion) was introduced by Sifneos to describe the condition of limited fantasy and emotional life. The Paris school of Marty and de M'Uzan had already described in 1963 a type of psychosomatic patient who was characterized by inability to fantasize freely, by *pensée opératoire* and by 'dreamless concretism'.

Limited perception of inner feelings and difficulty in communicating inner experience is particularly pronounced in psychosomatic patients. In this respect they differ considerably from neurotics, who are quite willing to talk about their ambivalent emotional lives. The manner of speech employed by neurotic patients also differs strongly from that of psychosomatic patients, who are frequently conspicuous by their poor vocabulary and inability to verbalize conflictual content.

Yet another difference between these two groups is that psychosomatic patients are well adjusted to their environment. They may deceive not only the people around them with an air of complacency but themselves as well, perhaps for several years. Even when they present with their symptoms at the doctor's they live under the delusion of having no emotional problems. For these patients, the language of the organs, pain, is the alarm signal emanating from their undisturbed identity with the world, as von Weizsäcker put it (quoted by Huebschmann 1952).

The origins of alexithymia are to be found in the type of family environment in which expression of feelings was out of place when confronted with the 'realities' of life. This tendency can then become more ingrained after many years of strenuous adjustment to social norms.

Although most authors agree about the core symptoms of this pattern of behaviour, the term 'alexithymia' is not without its critics, particularly with respect to its clinical implications. What seems important to us is that *the doctor should not suffer from alexithymia* if he wishes to treat psychosomatic patients!

Object Loss

Object loss is frequent in the initial stages of psychosomatic disease. Freyberger (1976) describes it as the occurrence of an actual, impending or imaginary loss. By object we understand animate and inanimate factors of the environment (i.e. persons too). A relationship exists between the subject and environmental factors that may assume the form of a strong attachment. A typical example of object loss is the absence of a person to whom the patient has become deeply attached. This is just as true for temporary or permanent loss of contact with, say, relatives as it is for being deprived of one's occupation.

Psychosomatic patients are not in a position to work through their object loss adequately. Owing to their labile feeling of self-esteem, it assumes the form of a narcissistic trauma, and the loss as such is not overcome. The sequel may be a form of depressive illness in which the patient is dominated by the giving up–given up complex (Engel and Schmale 1968). The depression may in turn be followed by physical disturbances. Using the work of von Engel and Schmale as his starting point, Freyberger (1976b) cites the following psychodynamic factors as being characteristic of psychosomatic patients:

1. Reactive depression after object loss and narcissistic trauma.
2. Oral regressive traits.
3. Defence against aggression.
4. Insufficient insight.

These he summarized under the heading 'disturbance in pregenital maturation' are intended – as is alexithymia – to describe the factors disposing to psychosomatic disease. On the basis of the terms 'alexithymia' and 'disturbance in pregenital maturation', Freyberger drew up his outline of psychosomatic development, which assigned the following keywords to the headings 'symptom', 'conflict' and 'personality':

Symptom

1. Emotional exhaustion.
2. Exhaustion depression.

Conflict

1. Object loss.
2. Narcissistic trauma.
3. Defence against aggression.

Personality Make-Up

1. Ego weakness, i.e. insufficient insight, injured 'primal trust', reduced frustration tolerance, increased dependency needs, very limited capacity for learning new emotional behaviour.
2. 'Emotional vacuum' owing to decreased awareness of feelings and the tendency to automatic thought processes, together with a reduced ability to work through problems emotionally due to an inadequate inner relationship to unconscious fantasies. Side by side with this characteristic is the compensatory trait of recounting physical sensations and hypochondriacal details.
3. Oral-narcissistic disorder with the marked tendency to experience object loss that cannot be worked through.
4. Defensive behaviour, particularly the complaining-cum-accusatory manner that implies a strong need for dependence on key figures, in order to win back objects involving disappointment and to compensate illness.

1.2.3 Models Based on the General-Systems Theory

Von Weizsäcker's introduction of the 'subject' into medicine revealed limits to thinking merely in terms of cause and effect. This acquired equal resonance with his description of reciprocal connections between the body and its environment in his concept of a gestalt cycle, known also as the morpho-psycho-physiological circle.

The situational circuit concept of von Uexküll is that an individual experiences and shapes his subjective world by interpretation (*Bedeutungsgebung*) and behaves accordingly (*Bedeutungsverwertung*). The psychosomatic reaction to it occurs when a corresponding, innermost readiness is present, a disposition that bears the hallmarks of a person's past.

Both approaches may be regarded as prototypes based on the general-systems theory. In recent times they have been of help in describing complex interactions significant to the development of psychosomatic illness.

It should be appreciated that the general-systems theory evolved from the natural sciences early this century and its applicational aspects did not make inroads into psychosocial and therapeutic fields of activity until the fifties. It was particularly in mathematics, physics and biology that a shift took place from a reductionist model such as that used by Newton and Darwin to a systemic paradigm that no longer tried to attribute the cause of a given phenomenon to a single factor but to the sequel of a summation of factors. Their *special interaction* alone finally enabled the phenomenon to arise. Einstein and Heisenberg were trail blazers of this new trend in the natural sciences.

The systemic concept views man as an open subsystem within a hierarchy of other open subsystems. This view was formulated more precisely by Gunthern, who attempted to include the individual in a systemic-holistic concept. He describes on the one hand the various levels of the human organism, namely, physiological, cognitive, emotional and transactional, while on the other he sees the individual as a personality both acting upon and being acted upon by sociocultural events of which it is part. Changes at one level of the organism, say, on the interactional plane, work as a stimulant in modifying processes taking place at other levels such as that of the somatic.

In his description of the human organism, von Bertalanffy developed a concept of hierarchical orders into which simpler systems (e.g. cells) are integrated as elements or subsystems within more complex systems. These in turn form part of even more complex systems (e.g. organisms) which interact on an advanced hierarchical plane with their environment and form social systems. This vista revived a principle put forward by von Ehrenfels at the close of the last century: a whole (a system) is greater than the summation of its parts (the subsystems). With increased complexity, systems evolve new properties absent at subsystem levels.

Language and procedures adequate for less complex systems often prove unsatisfactory in describing the phenomena under discussion. The solution remains elusive when attempts are made to reduce a newly formed complex such as a psychosomatic history to a biological context since the phenomenon loses its specific properties on reverting to a lower hierarchical plane of the system.

Incorporating the general-systems theory into the principles of treatment has helped evolve various schools of family therapy that no longer focus upon the individual but devote more attention to interactions between two or more persons. Thus even the way of looking at the causes of such problems has undergone sea change. The root of the trouble is no longer regarded as being the personality profile of the individual, with his or her psychodynamic response to past experience, feelings and dreams. The new approach to understanding the disorder is to study the behavioural facets of interaction in a multiple relationship frequently having its own covert codes. The multiple constellation presented by the family unit is thought of as a system ensuring equilibrium and defined by certain rules. This attitude has yet another far reaching consequence: the formulation of questions assessing guilt and cause may be modified. No longer does a sole individual bear the blame or is sick; the rules holding the family together as a system constitute the cause of the illness. The family unit thus becomes the target of diagnosis and treatment.

1.2.4 Sociopsychosomatics

The term 'sociopsychosomatics' was first introduced into the German literature by Schäfer (1966). Delius (1975) considered it to represent a pluralist approach to shedding light on pathogenesis. Emphasis is placed on social and interpersonal relationships and the conflicts arising from them that result in psychosomatic disease.

For Delius, sociopsychosomatic medicine begins when a patient who is concerned about his health, who feels ill or is ill, comes to realize in his interaction with the doctor and nursing staff that, by virtue of their frankness and sincerity, they are aware of his human and social problems.

Mitscherlich also regarded psychosomatics as social medicine since it attempted to identify – even if in a somewhat fragmentary fashion – pathogenic social situations in each individual case. Social interrelationships and constitutional factors receive especial attention in the published work of Wolff and Wolf. They emphasize the importance of the kind of situation prevailing at the time and corresponding cultural influences.

Over a period of many years at Cornell University, Hinkle carried out exemplary systematic investigations on populations of different origin, race and culture. His general conclusions were as follows:

1. On average, most illnesses occur in a small section of the total population.
2. Everyone shows a certain individual propensity towards illness, i.e. the mean frequency of illness remains constant. The sick become sicker, the healthy healthier.
3. The times of onset of illness are not evenly distributed; they are clustered around certain events, e.g. when certain processes in the environment are perceived as menacing, overtaxing, boding failure or in other ways conflictual.

Blohmke described the ramifications of sociopsychosomatics along the following lines:

Society in its broadest sense, including the environment, acts on the individual by directly influencing psychic processes. These trigger emotions that lead to biochemical reactions via the hypothalamus, sympathetic nervous system and the adrenals, which in turn affect the cardiovascular system and immunobiological response. The extent of these reactions on psychosocial factors is largely dependent on individual personality structure. Pronounced changes in emotional equilibrium go hand in hand with more frequent illness.

Labhardt points out in this connection that social and technical developments in recent years have led to a change in all norms. In the course of this social upheaval, tensions develop between the individual and his environment that are contributory factors in psychosomatic disease. This form of illness is a sequel to faulty development in the relations between different social structures.

A summary of the developments described is shown in Table 1.

Table 1. Summarizing the historical outline

From 1885	Freud: Conversion
1899	Pavlov: Influence of emotion on physiological processes
1912	Adler: Locus minoris resistentiae
1922	Deutsch: Organ neuroses
1934	Cannon: Emergency states
1943	Dunbar: Personality profiles
1946	Selye: Adaptation syndrome
1950	Alexander: Conflict specificity
1957	Hinkle, Wolff: Environmental factors
1963	von Uexküll: Differentiation of conversion disorders
1963	Marty, de M'Uzan: *Pensée opératoire*
1966	Schäfer: Sociopsychosomatics
1967	Engel: Object loss
1973	Sifneos, Nemiah: Alexithymia
1975	Bateson: General-systems theory
1981	Locke: Psychoneuroimmunology
1982	Maturana: Autopoietic systems
1985	Besedovsky: Proof of interaction between CNS and immune system.

1.2.5 Conclusion to the Precepts

It may be said in summary that psychosomatic medicine is not so much a specialized branch of medical science as an approach that takes into account the many different causes of illness. From this it should be clear that it covers a correspondingly wide area of research. Special interest, particularly in matters of research, is directed towards that specific group of disorders in which emotional factors play an important part. It is however eminently desirable that in losing its own distinct label psychosomatics should evolve into a way of thinking that might be called 'integral medicine'.

The theory of psychosomatic disease is based on numerous clinical observations that on the whole paint a convincing picture. The individual components that go to make up such disorders, however, can seldom be explained conclusively. Experimentally confirmed hypotheses are likewise rare.

The aim of research should therefore be to further the knowledge of psychosomatic correlates, given their importance. The World Health Organization has taken on the task of preparing a report on psychosomatic disorders and to this end has produced a list of the problems to which attention should be directed.This includes retrospective and prospective crossover studies, psychological tests, pathophysiological laboratory investigations, the study of innate behavioural tendencies, the psychophysiology of development, and the evaluation of therapeutic and epidemiological data.

At this juncture we should also consider the question of where to draw the line between psychosomatic disorders and illnesses of other origins. Here we touch on a delicate problem that throws into relief the contradiction inherent in the term 'psychosomatic'. To confine the use of this expression to certain quite specific disorders would be to reject the monistic concept of medicine; the dualism of mind and body would rise again like the phoenix from its ashes. One would be tempted to neglect psychic factors in certain disorders and somatic in others. The 1964 report of the WHO expert committee placed stress on this paradox but made no attempt to solve the problem. As far as the dividing line is concerned, the report states that this could be drawn in different places depending on whether one's prime interest is prophylaxis, therapy or research.

Siebeck summarized this paradox in his observation that while a distinction should be made between body, emotion and intellect, they should neither be fused nor separated.

Minkowski's view of this problem (quoted by Fain) is particularly enlightening: 'The combination of the two elements in each of the expressions "psychosomatic" and "somatopsychic" leaves something to be desired since it conjures up ideas of a dualism which in reality does not exist. A human being is a single entity, whether healthy or sick. There is simply no other way of putting it. In my opinion the essence of psychosomatic medicine lies not so much in the mere bringing together of psychic and somatic factors as in attempting to take a human being as he is, a living combination of body and mind.'

Definition

The term 'psychosomatic' as used in the following chapters includes a range of meanings which cannot be bracketed by a single definition. One aspect covers *psychosomatic disease*, which distinguishes between conversion symptoms, functional disturbances (organ neuroses) and the disease in the narrower sense of the word. Another aspect is *psychosomatic medicine*, a general approach that takes into account the complex somato-psychosocial interactions involved in the development of a disease, in particular their importance in structuring therapy.

2 Psychosomatic Disorders

Psychosomatic reactions occur in particularly stressful situations, for example: giddiness after a narrow escape, loss of appetite after bereavement, and even an amorous throbbing of the heart. Such symptoms usually disappear when the situation triggering the stimuli subsides. All types of people may experience psychosomatic *reactions*. Faulty emotional development is by no means an essential condition (Beck 1969).

Psychosomatic disorders are of a different character and may be split into the following main groups:

1. *Conversion Symptoms*: These are a secondary somatic response and working over of a neurotic conflict. The symptoms have a symbolic character and may be taken to represent an attempt to solve the conflict. Conversion symptoms generally relate to the voluntomotary and sensory organs. Examples are hysterical paralysis, paresthesia, psychogenic blindness and deafness, vomiting, and various sensations of pain.
2. *Functional Syndromes*: This group contains the major proportion of problem patients who consult their doctor with a shifting, often diffuse, spectrum of complaints. These may refer to the cardiovascular system, gastrointestinal tract, locomotor system, respiratory organs, or urogenital tract (see Table 2). The helplessness of the physician faced with this pattern of complaints is perhaps reflected by the great variety of terms. Functional disturbances involving individual organs or systems are present, but in most cases evidence of tissue damage is absent. Unlike conversion symptoms, the individual symptom has no specific significance, constituting merely a sequel to disturbed bodily function. Alexander (1951) considered such features to be signs that accompany affects and have no expressive character. He called them organ neuroses.

Table 2. Chief attendant symptoms of functional syndromes (based on von Uexküll)

Somatic	Psychic
globus	inner disquiet
paresthesia (mouth, tongue and extremities)	aprosexia, exhaustibility
impaired breathing	depression of mood
cardiac sensations	anxiety states
bouts of eructation	sleep disturbances

3. *Psychosomatic Disorders in the Narrower Sense (Psychosomatoses)*: Underlying these disorders is a primary physical reaction to a conflict situation or stress. Such a reaction is accompanied by morphologically demonstrable tissue lesions and objective organic findings. The choice of organ is influenced by a ready predisposition. This group includes the classic, 'holy seven' psychosomatic disorders:

Bronchial asthma,
ulcerative colitis,
essential hypertension,
neurodermatitis,
rheumatoid arthritis,
duodenal ulcer,
anorexia.

Other groupings are feasible such as those of Engel (1967, modified from Heim 1966a,b):

Psychogenic Disturbances (primary psychic phenomena with no or only imaginary involvement of the body):
Conversion symptoms;
hypochondriacal reactions;
reactions to psychopathological conditions.

Psychophysiological Disturbances (somatic reactions in the broadest sense triggered by psychic factors):
Physiological symptoms accompanying states of emotion and affective conditions;
organic disorders precipitated by emotional stress.

Psychosomatic Disorders in the Narrow Sense (somatopsychic-psychosomatic disturbances) with the following characteristics:
Onset at any age (more common in late adolescence);
once precipitated, their course may be chronic, simple or recurrent;
mental stress a determining factor, in most cases specific psychodynamic conditions for specific organic disorders; strikingly constant psychological traits.

Somatopsychic Disturbances:
Psychic reactions to somatic disorders.

2.1 Disorders of the Respiratory Organs

The first necessity facing a baby when it is separated from its mother's body is breathing. The first cry, which heralds the end of the state of apnea existing until birth, also represents the child's first expression of independent life.

The equating of breathing with autonomy is indelibly impressed on the body. That respiration is also connected with self-expression is suggested by the phrase 'to have an air of something', which has become rooted in our idiom. Indeed, breathing reflects and reveals emotional and affective processes, and does so more reliably than any other autonomically controlled function. Grief reduces the depth of respiration, while happiness increases it; anxious people have superficial and irregular breathing, and so on. Shakespeare was evidently aware of such correlations, for in *Macbeth* the doctor is asked if he can 'raze out the written troubles of the brain and . . . cleanse the stuffed bosom' of his patient.

2.1.1 Bronchial Asthma

Basic Aspects

Bronchial asthma is a disturbance in expiration and may occur at any age. Children under ten are particularly affected. The disorder has a close relationship with skin diseases (see Sect. 2.6 on allergy, pp. 77–79). A distinction is usually made between allergic (extrinsic) and non-allergic (intrinsic) asthma, the latter embracing reflex asthma and those forms precipitated by infection and exertion. Owing to the many different forms of asthma, the condition is frequently regarded as the 'somatic last lap' of various organic and emotional factors rather than as constituting a uniform clinical picture. One of the characteristics of bronchial asthma appears to be conditioning. It is thus possible that a patient who is allergic to flowers will also suffer an asthmatic attack on seeing artificial flowers. In such a case the attack is clearly triggered solely by the significance flowers have for the patient.

The asthmatic attack is frequently regarded as the equivalent of repressed weeping. Von Weizsäcker (1951) compares the attack to the screaming and crying of a child protesting loss of security; he views the episode as 'a scene of tears acted by the lungs'. The observation that an attack of bronchial asthma can be brought to an end by a bout of sobbing tends to support this interpretation. In many respects this disease bears a close relationship to migraine and allergic skin conditions, which can likewise be improved by weeping. Bräutigam and Christian (1973) attribute repressed weeping to patients being subjected to reproach and rejection in childhood when they cried for their mother.

The poets too have not failed to render their interpretions of the feelings inspired by the ability to breathe freely. In Talismane (Buch des Sängers) Goethe wrote:

Im Atemholen sind zweierlei Gnaden
Die Luft einziehen, sich ihrer entladen

Jenes bedrängt, dieses erfrischt;
So wunderbar ist das Leben gemischt.

(There are two graces in breathing: drawing in air and discharging it. The former constrains, the latter refreshes; so marvellously is life mixed. [Prose translation from: Goethe: Selected Classics. Edited by David Luke. Penguin Classics, London, 1986]).

Then there is that part of Beethoven's *Fidelio* where the prisoners rejoice on being freed from their chains:

Oh what joy to breathe freely
In the open air!
Up here alone is life!
The dungeon is a tomb.

(English translation and copyright: Lionel Salter; Deutsche Grammophon).

Personality Profile

A disturbed relation to the mother in early life generates conflict in the patient between the 'wish for tenderness' on the one hand and the 'fear of tenderness' on the other (de Boor 1965). According to Heim et al. (1970) the patient is characterized by underlying anxiety with hysterical and/or hypochondriacal traits. The patient himself is unaware of such anxiety. Bräutigam (1969) considered that 'in asthmatic attacks there was not only a retention of air but of feelings and emotions too'.

Von Weizsäcker (1951) and Fuchs (1965) see a correlation between disturbed respiratory function and the impaired ability of the patient to 'give and take'. Fuchs ascribed the condition to a kind of fear that developed into aggressive defensive tactics and tension that degenerated into compulsive acquisitiveness. This was the type of behavioural expression that came to a head during an asthmatic crisis, all inherent sense of composure being lost.

The conflicts in this 'give-and-take' aspect of the problem have also been described by Marty, who noted that in severe cases of allergy, patients had the tendency to identify themselves with those persons directly confronting them and to 'blend' with them, so to speak.

Treatment

Various psychotherapeutic techniques can complement correct somatic treatment very effectively indeed. Success depends to a very great extent on whether the conflict can be resolved between the marked anaclitic and defensive tendencies of the patient towards his doctor. Too much should not be expected of the patient in coping with feelings brought into play by both the proximity of the therapist and the dialogue. Petzold and Hahn reported on a patient's abrupt breakdown in psychological defenses resulting in psychotic symptoms (decompensation) that was presumably the sequel to radical intervention too near the mark. Such basic changes in syndromes have frequently been observed.

In respiratory treatment heavily orientated towards body therapies such as autogenic training and other relaxation techniques, the patient finds less opportunity to act out his own particular conflict with the therapist. Yet Fuchs saw other advantages in respiratory therapy. He considered that in breathing, the give-and-take process was – 'atmospherically' speaking – uninterrupted even if easily disturbed. Should it be possible to revive this rhythmic interplay once it has been thrown into disorder by anxiety or agitation, a positive influence will be exerted internally just as inner conditions are reflected externally. There will be no precipitate restoration of the desired harmony, but the path will be cleared for relaxing, relinquishing and opening up.

Deter reported on outpatient treatment of asthmatics in illness-orientated group therapy using these guidelines:

1. Giving information on the pathology and therapy relating to the various types of asthma. Guidance and instruction about the disorder – for a variety of reasons often inadequate – are aimed on the one hand at dispelling the patient's fear and on the other at motivating him to cope with the illness.
2. Training for safe and suitable codes of behaviour. The multifactorial nature of asthmatic attacks makes this very important since any emotional symptoms will promote inappropriate reactions. Such symptoms tend to be particularly marked in this illness, an example being excessive anxiety or its denial.
3. Teaching relaxation and breathing techniques. This will complement medication and allow the patient either to obtain relief from respiratory distress by himself or, in an emergency, to keep it in check until such time as a doctor or hospital can be contacted.
4. Open discussion within the group. This enables patients to exchange ideas and personal experiences and gain a feeling of security.
5. Promoting group interaction. This can acquire a certain degree of self-dynamism and lead to an emotional discussion between the members of the group and its leaders. It then falls to the therapist to verbalize in part the unconscious processes present and contribute to the self-analysis of patients.

Used to supplement standard internal treatment, the above can improve bodily, emotional, and social well-being, which in turn make considerable reductions in medication possible. Some discrimination must nevertheless be observed regarding indications: while middle-aged patients with much emotional trouble or severe somatic symptoms may benefit both physically and emotionally from illness-orientated group therapy, it is not indicated for older patients with counterphobic traits or for those with impaired pulmonary function. Whether young patients with mild asthma benefit from this group therapy only when the illness has developed, or need another type of psychotherapy, has at this writing not been determined.

2.1.2 Coughing and Singultus

The primary purpose of coughing is to clear the respiratory tract of foreign bodies and attendant irritations. It is related to vomiting, the digestive equivalent of the same process. Oppressive emotions can promote bronchial secretion just as they can stimulate gastric secretion. Coughs that are initially of organic origin but are reinforced and maintained without expectoration are indicative of inner tension. The coughing then serves as a relief. It can also embody an attempt to get rid of inner desires that are felt to be alien and dangerous. The expectorate is an even clearer expression of disgust or hostility, being next to excrement in the repertoire of insults.

The cause underlying a chronic cough is frequently a feeling of anger or fury that the patient does not feel capable of expressing in words. Jores (1976) speaks of 'protest coughing'. The protest is usually directed against a specific person well within the reach of the conscious mind. This author describes how he asked a patient in German '*wem wollen Sie etwas husten?*' – who do you want to give a piece of your mind to? But in order to understand the significance of the idiom, it must be realized that the German verb *husten* means 'to cough' (the colloquial expression in English 'to cough up' represents a parallel in idiomatic usage but means of course something quite different). The point here is that Jores' patient reacted quickly to the question and realized the connection between his repressed aggression and the cough. The patient should be encouraged in the course of the therapeutic communication to formulate his protest in words or to change by other means the underlying situation. Supplementary respiratory therapy or autogenic training may also be of value.

Singultus, an inspiratory disorder, is frequently seen in children exposed to unpredictable oscillation between extreme generosity and punitive severity on the part of the parents who do not really have love to give them. The attacks occur following a deterioration in this situation or as a result of insecurity (Bridge et al. quoted from Rubin & Mandell 1966).

2.1.3 The Nervous Breathing Syndrome

This term covers various forms of respiratory disorders such as deep sighing respiration, hyperventilation and what is known as 'respiratory corset'.

Deep sighing respirations are characterized by prolonged, audible breathing at maximal depth repeated at frequent intervals. Christian et al. (1965) consider this kind of respiration to be the expression of nervous, ill-humoured exhaustion after fruitless efforts and disappointment.

In hyperventilation the patient inspires more air than he needs. It resembles the type of breathing that normally accompanies physical exertion, and may be either acute or chronic. The cause is emotional tension with underlying anxiety. Protracted hyperventilation indicates anxiety neurosis (Weimann 1968).

'Respiratory corset' describes the symptom of not being able to breath deeply. It frequently accompanies cardiac symptoms and occurs mainly in patients having obsessive-compulsive personality structures and is a sign of inhibited expression (Jores 1976).

2.1.4 The Hyperventilation Syndrome

Basic Aspects

The hyperventilation syndrome is an emotional disorder in which rapid deep breathing – often unnoticed by the patient – is accompanied by air hunger and a feeling of tightness in the chest. Anginoid symptoms, and abdominal pain usually associated with aerophagia, meteorism, and flatulence, round off in many cases the clinical profile.

Marked symptoms of tetany with sharp flexion of the extremities (carpopedal spasm) tend to be rare, while complaints of burning and prickling sensations in the oral region are frequent.

Attacks develop without any organic or endocrinological basis. Although they are of emotional origin in over 90% of cases, organic differential diagnosis must be considered (e.g. tetanus, encephalitis, tumours, etc.).

Rose (1976) views normocalcemic tetany separately since the term 'hyperventilation syndrome' does not do justice to the specificity of the attacks and the deep-seated neurotic personality disorders of such tetany patients.

Lewis (1957) describes the circular, self-reinforcement of the hyperventilation syndrome, in which not only anxiety leads to hyperventilation, but the symptom pattern strengthens and lengthens hyperventilation, bringing about a vicious circle (see Fig. 1).

Women are affected about three times more frequently than men. With increasing age symptoms become rarer in both sexes.

Personality Profile

The patients usually exhibit marked character traits. Their basic attitude is one of anxiety depression with hypochondriacal and phobic features. They frequently put up a false front to hide their latent fears. Extremely conscious of social norms, they give the impression of being pleasant, conscientious and adaptive patients. They are accustomed to putting their own requirements last.

These patients are strongly inhibited in their expressive behavioural patterns and particularly incapable of experiencing and working through

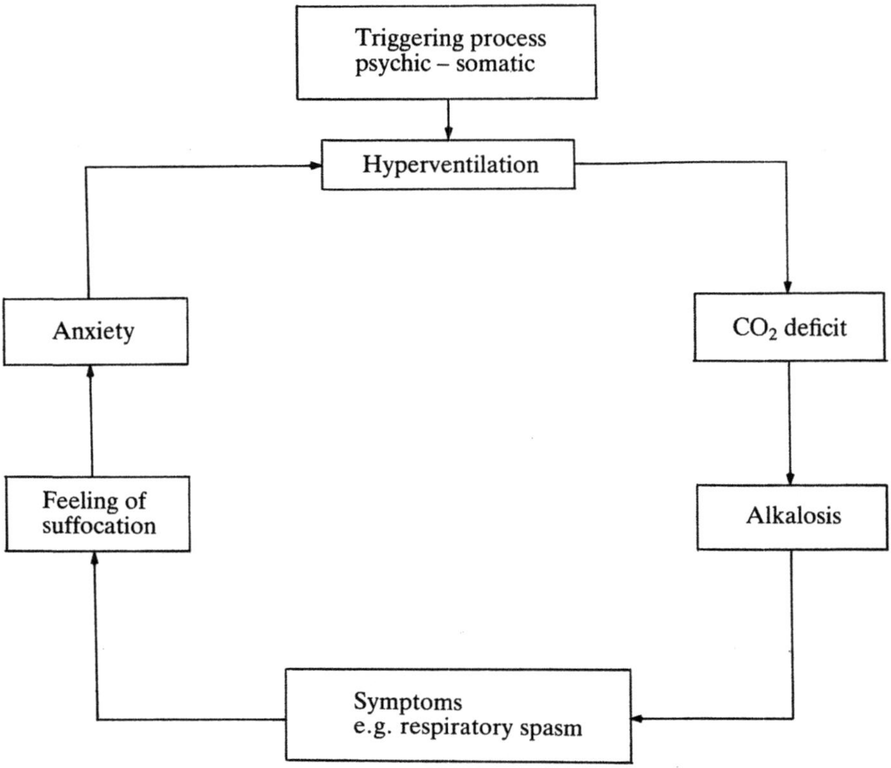

Fig. 1. Self-reinforcement of the hyperventilation syndrome (modified after Klussmann 1986)

aggressive instinctual impulses. They usually describe themselves as having pent-up feelings or that they passively 'swallow too much'. This tendency to accept unreasonable demands imposed on them and the inability to assert themselves are not infrequently experienced as oppressive (Rose 1976).

Another tendency is to become dependent on a dominant partner. This forms a continuity with childhood patterns. According to Bach (1969), the patients come mainly from families in which they were brought up by quite considerate but frustrating parents, in a heavily norm orientated and anti-individualistic atmosphere hardly suitable for children. The stronger bond was generally with the weaker parent since this presented a relatively better opportunity for an emotional relationship. Aggressive emotions against the dominant parent were mostly repressed because they were felt to incur existential hazards. Rose goes on to say that experience showed it was better to live with a far stronger partner, even if the price paid for security involves continually shelving one's own desires and requirements. And even if the partner's behaviour is offensive or frustrating, no protest is uttered since it is deemed pointless. The life patterns of these patients show that they repeatedly place themselves in situations of dependency in which they have less and less to say, and at the same time experience crippling anxiety at the thought of losing such ambivalent persons of reference.

The conflict situation precipitating the attacks contains on the one hand elements of real or imaginary frustration or illness, and, on the other, fear of losing the security provided by dependency. The attacks occur not infrequently after situations demanding outwardly self-assertive and aggressive action, of which the patient is incapable on account of his general feeling of helplessness and fear of losing the protection previously described.

Treatment

Treatment is aimed at interrupting the attack by rebreathing expired air. After alkalization of the blood by the lowered CO_2 levels during hyperventilation a feedback is thus achieved. This has a calming effect on patients, some of whom experience annihilation anxiety as a result of the attacks. They learn that their health or life is not endangered. At the same time, rebreathing offers the patient a therapy paving the way to self-regulation. Of no mean importance is the feeling this gives him of being able to master the symptoms he once felt powerless to oppose. Underlying conflicts that have not been resolved can be tackled on a long-term basis by modified psychoanalytic techniques. The physical manifestation of unconscious aggressive impulses during the attacks would suggest the additional applicability of body therapies ranging from relaxation, physiotherapy and a new kind of psychosomatic training with music. The aim is improved perception of the intrapersonal sphere.

2.1.5 Pulmonary Tuberculosis

Basic Aspects

Only a small proportion of persons infected by a potential pathogen become clinically ill. This is just as true for tuberculosis, which is transmitted by droplet or dustborne infections, as it is for illnesses occasioned by other germs (e.g. meningococci) that can, but do not inevitably, result in the outbreak of an infectious disease. The body's resistance appears to involve a close connection between personality variables and stress on the one hand and the reaction of the immune system on the other. The relatively young but rapidly developing discipline of *psychoneuroimmunology* will certainly provide interesting data in coming years on questions of resistance and susceptibility to infection.

In tuberculosis there is a striking discrepancy between infection and disease actually associated with morbidity: almost every adult has at some time in his life been subject to invasion by tubercle bacilli. A study in Switzerland showed that 80% of those taking part reacted positively to tuberculin by the age of forty, but only 5–10% of those infected had active progressive disease. A pathological concordance rate of about 50% for identical twins and 25% for dissimilar twins suggests a genetic disposition.

Personality Profile

As early as 1826 the French internist Laennec described what he saw as the situation leading to pulmonary tuberculosis in the following words: '*les passions tristes, profondes et de longue durée*'. The long duration of these deep-seated emotional states is also considered important in modern psychosomatics. For it is not so much the quirks of fortune and emotional traumas that have pathogenetic significance as *chronic* conditions. An example would be when the choice of an occupation or marriage partner hangs in the balance. Continuously trying tension and conflict, disappointments, incessant fear and an unbalanced personality may influence the onset of illness. In one of his publications, Huebschmann refers to case histories reported by Stern providing convincing evidence of the disease constituting the equivalent of a vital decision. This material suggests that the patient recovers when an external decision is made, the internal decision in favour of illness then becoming superfluous.

Tuberculosis patients do not exhibit any uniform type of personality but they do have one trait in common – extreme vulnerability to any withdrawal of love coupled with the need to remain close to the mother in the safety zone surrounding her. While one type of patient will openly manifest his need for love, another would give anything to get away from this passive security although he has the same anxious need of it.

Treatment

In addition to prescribing chemotherapy and possibly surgical procedures it is important to take into account the patient's personality. The Dutch specialist Bronkhorst succeeded in showing that in more than half of the cases he studied cavitary lesions healed spontaneously when there was a good doctor-patient relationship and individual medical guidance. According to Kissen the pulmonary lesion can only heal if the emotional wound also does so.

The treatment indicated in hospitals and sanatoria is frequently rather a supportive, personal form of therapy centred around the patient's conflicts. After being discharged, many patients require continued psychotherapy in order to adapt to separation from the protective environment of the sanatorium and to receive support for the difficult problem of social reintegration. Some people believe, therefore, that in the interests of therapeutic stability, modern medical or surgical measures should only be applied in a psychosomatic context, in other words, together with supplementary psychotherapy.

2.2 Cardiovascular Disorders

The activity of the heart and emotional experience are very closely related. This is mirrored in everyday expressions and idiom: someone's heart leaps for joy or sinks into his boots, we can be hearty or heartless, lose heart, or the heart can 'stand still' with fear.

As far back as classical times the heart was held to be the seat of emotion and passion. The atomists thought anger came from the heart. Similarly, Plato considered the region between the throat and diaphragm to house wrath, bravery and love of honour. He also saw the heart to be a kind of alarm centre that issued a warning against evil designs on the body, whether they came from outside or were nurtured in the innermost desires. These ideas bear a certain resemblance to Freud's later theory of anxiety.

Mayer obtained scientific evidence of this relationship. In the course of his evaluations on heart-rate recordings over long periods, he became convinced that they contained a kind of psychoautonomic imprint, the characteristic features of which were in his opinion determined before birth. He reported further on a Heidelberg gynecologist who maintained that his many years of experience in this field enabled him to identify a given individual from readings taken in monitoring the fetal heart rate.

The heart is regulated by a profuse and complex supply of nerves. Neurovegetative dysequilibrium, to which anxious and particularly younger people are predisposed, tends strongly to act on the heart. In the absence of organic evidence, one speaks of functional heart disorders.

Heart complaints with no organic cause have been accorded a multiplicity of terms, which may in some measure reflect the great need on the part of the physician to find his bearings in dealing with such disorders. The compilation in Table 3 is by no means complete and thus but a sketchy guide for

Table 3. Selection of terminology sometimes used synonymously for anxiety symptoms relating to cardiac complaints. (After Nutzinger et al. 1987)

nervous palpitations	Hope 1832; Williams 1836
nervous heartbeats	Stokes 1855
inframammary pain	Coote 1858; Inman 1858
heart neurosis	Friedrich 1867
hyperkinesis cordis	Oppolzer 1867
irritable heart	McLean 1867; Da Costa 1871
neurasthenia	Beard 1880
anxiety neurosis	Freud 1895
neurocirculatory asthenia	Oppenheimer et al. 1918
effort syndrome	Lewis 1918
cardiac neurosis	Hamburger 1915; Schnur 1939; Caughey 1939
Da Costa's Syndrome	Wood 1941
functional cardiovascular disease	Friedmann 1947
anxiety reaction	American Psychiatric Association 1952
cardiac hypochondria	Bräutigam 1956
cardiophobia	Kuhlenkampff and Bauer 1960
functional cardiovascular syndrome	von Uexküll 1962

practitioner and clinician alike. In making a diagnosis, certitude regarding somatic findings is of course essential. Particularly in middle-aged patients it is no easy matter without an accurate history to distinguish, for example, an attack brought on by anxiety from one having the classic symptoms of angina pectoris. Positive psychopathological findings must thus substantiate an independent psychogenic basis for the symptoms.

In the differential diagnosis of functional cardiac disorders we distinguish between the following clinical pictures (Kröger et al. 1985a,b):

- Phobic (Type A) and contraphobic (Type B) cardiac neuroses,
- the hyperkinetic cardiac syndrome,
- paroxysmal supraventricular tachycardia.

2.2.1 Functional Heart Disorders

Cardiac Neurosis

Freud, who was familiar with these symptoms from his own experience, described them thus: disturbances in cardiac activity involving tachycardia, palpitations, cardiospasm and brief arrhythmias; respiratory disturbances (nervous dyspnea, asthma-like attacks), bouts of sweating, tremor, bulimia, dizziness, congestion, paresthesia.

Parade outlines the symptoms of cor nervosum as follows:

Cardiac Sensations
palpitations, tachycardia, hyperkinesis cordis, dysrhythmia, angina pectoris; anxiety, oppression, unrest, fear of death, depression.

Self-Observation
tendency to cling, fear of separation.

Nervous Dyspnea
hyperventilation, gasping for breath
fear of suffocation
paresthesias.

Autonomic Symptoms
'autonomic decompensation'
confusing variety of symptoms of attack
impaired physical endurance.

Under the collective term cardiac neurosis, Richter and Beckmann originally included any disturbance that made a patient consult a physician about heart complaints not originating from a physical illness. However, the criterion 'organically unaccountable' is sadly in need of extension.

Cardiac neurosis can be subdivided into groups differing primarily in the form taken by anxiety defence mechanisms:

Patients with the phobic form of cardiac neurosis constitute a rather homogenous group (Type A personalities). They are conspicuous in the doctor–patient relationship by their anaclitic need to keep seeking medical aid, and by their constant fear of death by heart failure. In the forefront of the psychodynamic picture is ambivalence towards separation: the incompatibility of the desire for separation and the dread of it.

The group of patients comprising the so-called Type B personalities, however, is far more heterogenous. In addition to the contraphobic form adopted by the complaint, it includes patients with strong hypochondriac-depressive constituents as well as those whose normally slight symptoms occur within the context of a depressive syndrome. As far as the psychodynamics are concerned, this group of patients exhibits in a similar manner the basic problem common to all cases of cardiac neurosis – ambivalence towards separation. A distinct difference with the phobic group lies in the way of coping with anxiety. In all their personal contacts, including the doctor–patient relationship, contraphobic patients try to preserve an image of fortitude and equanimity.

An important diagnostic criterion for cardiac neurosis of the phobic type is predictable commencement of the complaint pattern with a sympathicovasal sort of attack triggered by concurrent somatic and psychic factors leading to the characteristic vicious circle 'fear of fear' (Bergmann and Hahn).

Typical features of the attack are fast heart rate, raised blood pressure, giddiness, a feeling of weakness, bouts of sweating, and the characteristic fear of death. It may occur spontaneously, often in the morning at work after too little sleep.

Hahn et al. showed that the classic differentiation of these two types of cardiac neurosis may be found in this context, but if not, certainly in psychotherapeutic outpatient treatment. Findings were sparse in patients first seeking help in cardiological outpatient departments, not only findings regarding psychodynamic aspects of personality, but also those related to the initial sympathicovasal crisis. These patients thus appeared either to be in little need of therapy or responded well to somatic treatment.

The Hyperkinetic Heart Syndrome

This syndrome elicits vague cardiac complaints and many concomitant autonomic symptoms. The patients feel weak, their abilities ebb, and some become aware of higher pulse rates. Unlike the phobic form of cardiac neurosis, however, anxiety is rare and fear of death even more seldom.

Clinical findings include sinus tachycardia, often hypertension, increased cardiac output and reduced peripheral resistance. Since symptoms of the hyperkinetic heart syndrome largely reflect the pharmacological effects of catecholamine on β-receptors, β-blockers may be given after excluding hyperthyroidism to confirm the diagnosis ex juvantibus.

Besides their general apathy and tiredness, patients are conspicuous by their characteristic inhibition of motor aggressive drives. As children they were often very lively and outgoing, and it was not until puberty that this reserve developed. Symptoms first seem to appear when they are pressured to develop behaviour patterns over and above their habitual circumstances and aptitudes.

Paroxysmal Supraventricular Tachycardia

While with cardiac neurosis and hyperkinetic heart syndrome it is possible to start out with the idea of the disturbances being psychogenic, this heart condition constitutes an excellent example of what happens when physiogenic and psychogenic stress factors arise simultaneously and complement one another. In paroxysmal supraventricular tachycardia there exists a predisposition to attacks owing to peculiarities in the autonomic innervation of the auricles.

Though harmless enough on their own, supraventricular and ventricular extrasystoles together with emotional strain can eventually release the whole pattern of symptoms.

From a psychodynamic angle, patients are characterised by severe emotional inhibition causing them sometimes to appear over-compliant, even equable and calm as far as the practitioner is concerned. Yet the complete personality profile is shown to contain a hidden, repressed enmity, which eventually comes to light, revealing occasional aggressive outbursts.

Treatment

Statistical investigations confirm that the probability of these patients dying of heart disease or contracting a somatic cardiac disorder is if anything lower and not, as one might expect, higher than for a random sample of the population.

Patients with functional cardiac disorders are by no means malingerers. They suffer intensely from their symptoms, particularly when afflicted by thoroughgoing paroxysmal tachycardia, dyspnea and a sensation of constriction of the chest. Should the doctor inform them that their complaint is 'only' of nervous origin, they may gain the impression that inadequate respect has been paid to both their symptoms and to their personality.

First and foremost the patient should be assured that his heart is organically in order, the prognosis good, and that the disturbances are of a functional nature. When this explanation (possibly in conjunction with symptomatic treatment such as sedatives and β-blockers in low doses) proves of little help and no improvement is noted, some form of psychotherapy is indicated. This combined with drug treatment or physiotherapy is of benefit only when the patient has learned to perceive and work over the situational and conflictual components of his illness and is capable of abandoning his bodily orientated, rather over-protective attitude by reducing anxiety.

Symptomatic treatment without a specific indication in view can indeed aggravate the complaint; in their conflictual situation, patients may feel they have been misunderstood and, consciously or unconsciously, respond either with a change or an increase in the original symptoms. The frequent tendency of such patients to transfer their attentions to those practising fringe or unorthodox medicine can be avoided only by using sympathy and understanding in talks that establish a contact. Once a trustful relationship has been built up, the long-term support often needed may be taken over by the general practitioner.

Should the relief afforded the patient prove inadequate, focal psychotherapy centred around the conflict is then indicated, or even one of the rather time-consuming individual, group or family therapies (Hahn 1965; Hahn et al. 1973).

2.2.2 Coronary Heart Disease

Basic Aspects

The number of deaths from infarction in the Federal Republic of Germany rose from 74,000 to 139,000 during the period extending from 1966 to 1976. This steep trend contrasted with the situation in the United States, where the mortality from cardiovascular disease receded by 13.2% during the years 1970 to 1975. For the corresponding period, the mortality rate in West Germany increased by 13.5%. According to data from the WHO infarction register established in Heidelberg, the annual rate in men under 50-years of age has in the meantime also fallen, in the 50–60 year-old group remained almost constant, and risen slightly in the 60–65 group (Bergdolt et al.). This differentiation within the age groups is similar to that in the United States, where the falling trend in infarction also began in the younger, then continued in older age groups.

Since the Heidelberg data are representative for about two-thirds of the population of West Germany, it may be assumed from the trend in and around this city that mortality rates for the disease are on the decline throughout the whole country.

The positive developments in the United States are apparently the result of extensive health education programmes on the risk factors of infarction, and it is a matter of great urgency that the German authorities should follow suit (Schettler and Greten).

Large-scale studies have established that the somatic risk factors include raised serum cholesterol levels, hypertension, diabetes mellitus, obesity, tobacco abuse and lack of exercise. The cumulative effect determines the somatic risk factor, which is increased by socioecological and psychological factors.

There is however little point in considering individual factors. Although somatic factors strongly increase the risk of infarction, accurate prognosis can be made only after psychic factors have been taken into account. Present attempts to determine the risk of infarction employ a multifactorial approach: both the measurable somatic risk factors and those components of the personality structure predisposing the patient to infarction must be regarded as a compromising entity. On the whole, it would appear that the constellation of hazards is so different for each individual that it is not possible to work out a uniform risk profile for all those endangered by coronary heart disease (Hahn 1971).

In this context, Christian et al. (1966) coined the term 'personality' at risk'. Its criteria are personality traits and environmental factors that together with organic risk factors are of consequence in deciding on causal relationships. In the opinion of Hahn et al.; coronary occlusion and thrombosis are almost invariably the result of the interdependent and cumulative effects of risk factors during the course of a chronic development frequently extending over many years, the onset of the actual illness being triggered off by an event of acute nature.

Personality Profile

Christian comments how it has long been accepted that the personality structure of patients at risk of infarction is different from that of 'neurotics'. Personalities at risk of infarction do not have the inhibited, emotionally labile and insecure traits of people all too emotionally conscious of illness. They do not, on the other hand, enjoy a state of psychological balance; their behaviour has been overadapted to a performance-orientated society and manifests rigid and compulsive traits.

The same author refers to the WHO studies in Heidelberg, which conclude that infarction patients conform too drastically to social norms, i.e. they are outwardly open and sociable but at the same time manifest quite contrary attitudes, particularly those of anxiety coupled with a degree of rigidity in their general behaviour.

According to Freyberger, the infarct patient's aspirations to high standards are only partly innate. The rest arise from a neurotic maladjustment and serve as a compensation. When the psychic predispositions so far described coincide with specific environmental situations, there is an increased risk of infarction from the psychosomatic aspect provided a measure of 'somatic compliance' is present in the form of a latent or manifest coronary insufficiency. The precipitative environmental situations that have their impact on the given psychic disposition and bring infarction in their wake frequently imply an experience of *object loss*.

Disappointments in personal relationships strongly suggesting a *separation*, as well as an occupational failure with distinct emotional *loss* components, constitute a particularly high emotional hazard for potential cases of infarction if a simultaneous narcissistic disorder is present.

The narcissistic disorder is the prime condition for inadequate 'working through' of an object loss. The outcome is a labilization of emotional states of inner security and well-being, a kind of 'labile self-awareness' showing distinct depressive features. Whether manifest or masked, this state of 'labile self-awareness' is evidenced in potential cases of infarction characterized by these psychodynamic processes. Labile self-awareness, which is sometimes manifested as a feeling of inferiority, thus constitutes an important inner motive for aspiring to high standards since the patient can build up a more or less stable pseudo-self-confidence by such compensatory means (Freyberger 1976a).

Schäfer (1976) distinguishes between two factors determining the risk of infarction: one is sclerosis and the other stress. Exacerbation of these factors may be caused by bad habits with regard to eating, drinking, smoking and exercise, as well as states of anxiety, tension, aggressivity and compulsion, which in turn may produce behaviour pregnant with risks. Blohmke aptly pointed out that here it is never a question of objectively operative factors but rather of the patient's subjective experience.

Rosenman and Friedman, Dunbar, Jenkins, and several other authors, have described behavioural patterns predisposing to coronary disease. Persons constantly aspiring to achieve something are particularly endangered. Haste, impatience, restlessness, constantly tensed facial muscles, the feeling of being pressed for time and bearing responsibility hallmark the patient at risk. Such patients tend to identify themselves so closely with their work that they have no time for anything else. They have an obsessive passion for work. Petzold's (1978) explanation for this is that the patients get along better in the performance-orientated sphere of work than they do in personal and family circles, finding such human proximity rather oppressive.

Then there is the marked tendency of these patients to overtax themselves. Jenkins, for example, has pointed out that they are often inadequately trained for their work. According to this, the risk of infarction should be greater for those 'on their way up' than for those already enjoying success and status. Patients at risk attempt to solve the conflictual situation arising from overstrain as they do for all conflicts: they call on themselves to be even quicker, stronger, and to achieve higher standards of perfection.

To such patients the fear that their efforts will end in failure is almost unthinkable and is carefully concealed behind a façade of impressive industry.

Roseman and Friedman (1959) described behaviour incurring the risk of coronary disease as Type A, a behavioural pattern with which such patients, by virtue of their personal traits, respond to situational challenges. The authors contrasted it with Type B behaviour, which occupies the opposite pole on the behavioural scale.

Type A and Type B characteristics are observable facets of behaviour, constituting in themselves neither risk factors nor a possible causal explanation of coronary disease.

Petzold (1976) points out that even a person with Type A behaviour may find creative calm, but tend to brood when things go wrong, progressively increasing inner tension until the way is paved for behaviour typical of the patient heading for cardiac infarction.

Treatment

The difficulties in treating patients with coronary disease are only too obvious from their personality structure. From the doctor's point of view the problem is to recognize the patient's aspirations to high standards as being a conflict situation. Efficiency and performance-orientation are only too readily equated with health: hard-working people are considered to be healthy.

Coronary patients tend to deny their conflicts. Freyberger speaks of a psychic scotomization. In candidates for infarction, this relates on the one hand to the constant overstrain produced by the inner urge for achievement and on the other to the marked health hazards in the form of tobacco abuse and increased calorie intake. Such denial is a defence mechanism that makes it very difficult to build up inner motivations for treatment.

Petzold (1976) makes basic distinctions between three types of treatment. Selection depends on aspects of personal development and the prevailing situation. The possibilities he advocates are as follows:

- individual counseling, information on behaviour conducive to health and special attention paid to cognitive processes;
- symptom-orientated body therapies (autogenic training, functional relaxation) without handling the problem of resistance;
- psychotherapy, including the handling of resistance and transference.

Psychotherapeutic follow-up of patients who have had an infarction is only indicated under the conditions described below:

1. The patient mentions a complaint that he feels he cannot overcome by himself and seeks the help of a doctor.
2. The doctor administering the treatment notices that the patient, despite his outward show of readiness, cannot follow repeated advice to change certain patterns of behaviour. This sort of advice is based on rational and scientific arguments.

In determining which type of psychotherapy is indicated, Petzold employs Degrecoustry's classification of infarction patients, which is as follows:

1. Impulsive patients.
2. Adapted patients.
3. Regressive patients.

Group activity in sport and exercise under medical supervision has proved of great value for impulsive patients. Such activities meet their motor needs.

A combination of group therapy and autogenic training is recommended for adapted patients.

The preferred treatment for regressive patients is psychotherapy since the troubles afflicting them may be apparent from their marked 'clinging' tendency or from depressive reactions.

In all cases of patients with coronary heart disease, detailed history taking is essential in order to elicit emotional disturbances and to find out how the patient deals with his innermost urges and feelings. The disturbances encountered vary greatly, and may include autonomic disorders of other organs, or emotional symptoms such as anxiety and compulsion.

2.2.3 Essential Hypertension

Basic Aspects

Recent research has had an increasing tendency to regard high blood pressure as a nonspecific biological signal, rather like abnormal erythrocyte sedimentation rates or fever, which may have many varied primary causes. In a review written in 1977, Weiner accordingly described essential hypertension as a non-uniform clinical picture that can arise owing to quantitative changes in various influences. In addition to somatic, there are social and psychic factors that are of different significance with regard to etiology, pathogenesis, and chronicity.

In the Federal Republic of Germany it was found that over 79% of 30–69-year-old men and 63% of women in the same age group were hypertensive and had blood pressures under inadequate medical control (Stieber et al.). On an average, hypertensive patients consult their general practitioner 8.5 times a year, i.e. twice as frequently as normotensive patients. This can be a pointer to already existing cardiovascular sequelae, which may in turn also reflect problems of management as well as the attitude of these patients towards drug therapy.

Hypertension has been recognized to be a risk factor of central importance, and medical antihypertensive therapy has clearly lowered morbidity and mortality rates. Nevertheless, important problems remain unsolved concerning the origin, development, and chronic tendencies of high blood pressure. The broadening of research by the inclusion of psychological and sociological aspects has improved understanding of factors influencing the illness and brought the basic methods of treatment up to optimal levels.

Table 4. The various forms of hypertension and their frequency (after Bernsheimer)

Form	%
Essential hypertension	79.9
Renal hypertension	14.0
Endocrine hypertension	3.5
Cardiovascular hypertension	2.0
Neurogenic hypertension	0.6

Bernsheimer listed the frequency and causes of the various forms of hypertension. The results are given in Table 4.

In 1982 von Uexküll described situational hypertension as the linking of specific conditions in the patient's milieu with blood pressure reactions. When there is a dispostion to react in this manner, environmental influences can trigger raised blood pressure. Such a disposition is individually shaped by the patient's past. Depending on the magnitude, duration and frequency of the vasoconstrictor reaction, situational changes in blood pressure during the early stages of hypertension appear to constitute increased risk of the condition becoming established. Together with shifts in baroreceptor values and changes in salt/water excretion by the kidneys, structural changes in the precapillaries lead to a fixed high blood pressure. Even if these changes are reversible in their early stages by medication and not morphologically permanent owing to connective tissue deposits in vessels where there is resistance to blood flow, epidemiological data nevertheless tend to confirm that people with a highly labile systolic blood pressure or oversensitive blood-pressure response are at greater risk of developing hypertension or coronary heart disease than normotensives (Schmidt).

Personality Profile

In discussing the personality of the hypertensive patient, frequent reference has been made to the intrapersonal conflict between aggressive impulses on the one hand and feelings of dependency on the other. Alexander (1951) described how hypertension was linked with the desire to give outward expression to enmity while at the same time there was a need for passive and adapted behaviour. His studies were followed by many others dealing with the personality structure of these patients. Their social behaviour is summed up as being over-adapted, tractable, performance orientated, passive, with a tendency to avoid conflict; it is further marked by restraint in both positive and negative affect.

While these patterns evidenced by earlier studies primarily relate to observable behaviour in patients, more recent investigations have shown that their perception of conflict and stress is also altered as against normotensives. In a study on health changes in air traffic controllers, Rose et al. showed that not only were those at risk who identified themselves too strongly with the job and were extremely sociable and adapted, but also those who refused to acknowledge the stress involved.

Baer et al. turned their attention to indirect familial interaction by investigating the conflictual behaviour in families with hypertensive fathers. They saw the family as a clinical unit and used a general-systems approach in setting up the following hypotheses:

The personality structure of a family member – e.g. the conflict of aggressive impulse and dependency of the hypertensive – affects the interaction of the whole family.

From the aspect of family dynamics, the following points regarding build-up of essential hypertension suggested themselves to the authors on conclusion of the study:

In every family certain rules evolve between parents and children for coping with conflicts. In families with hypertensive fathers, the children learn less effective ways of coping and finding solutions. This is shown by the predominance of negative, nonverbal communication in such families, e.g. not answering, turning away, and avoiding eye-to-eye contact. A variety of studies indicate that limited perception of conflict and stress, and conflict avoidance, correlate with the onset of high blood pressure. Such patterns of behaviour are thus acquired by children in the socialisation process of the family with the hypertensive father. While genetic aspects must be borne in mind, this approach could open up a complementary avenue of thought for the possible reduplication of essential hypertension.

The family pattern of interaction appears to be further marked by a kind of ban on communication that extends even to averbal means; taking in, observing, controlling and restraining activities tend to crowd out those that are of a yielding, informative, or participating nature (Kröger and Petzold).

Treatment

The doctor-patient relationship is frequently typified by the patient's aggressivity/dependence conflict. This reflects the scepsis and negative attitudes of this group of patients towards the doctor's proffered therapy and may result in their avoiding medical treatment or in drug defaulting. However, if the doctor-patient relationship and compliance are to run smoothly it would seem that not only does the personality structure of the individual patient play a role but also the interaction of the entire family. The family must, for example, be willing to work together with the doctor in questions of diet and compliance. The circumstances existing in treating hypertensive patients may be summed up as follows:

- Low motivation since subjective complaints are usually insignificant;
- effective medication possible;

personality factors dominated by an aggressivity/dependence conflict leading to possible tension in doctor-patient relations and expressed primarily in drug defaulting.

Early involvement of the social milieu is recommended as supplementary therapy. This may include a non-directive doctor-patient relationship, which does not activate the aggressivity/dependence conflict, an informatory attitude on the part of the doctor, reinforcement of the patient's self-responsibility and independence, as well as of self-perception (e.g. by measuring his own blood pressure). Naturally, the simplest possible dosage scheme should be prescribed.

Psychotherapy in addition to medication is indicated only if complaints are evident that are emotional in nature. On the whole, behavioural therapy and relaxation techniques prove quite valuable in complementing medication since less drug treatment may be needed when they are employed.

2.3 Aspects of Eating Behaviour

2.3.1 Nutrition

Eating habits mirror one's affective needs and current state of mental health, while exerting in turn their influence on these psychic aspects. Nor should it be overlooked that nourishment is often identified with love, as exemplified by numerous colloquial expressions. There is a kernal of truth in the saying 'the way to a man's heart is through his stomach', while 'I could eat you' is an expression of great affection. We also speak of being 'hungry for love', and our mouths remain in the service of tenderness and love throughout our lives. This link between the tender passions and nourishment goes back to an early phase in our development.

Nutrition as a Primary Experience

In the initial stages of life no other vital function plays such an important part in development as eating. The satisfaction of hunger produces a feeling of security and well-being. The child experiences the first relief from physical discomfort during nursing, and contact with the smooth, maternal skin gives him the feeling of being loved. The infant also experiences the pleasurable sensations in the mouth, lips and tongue while being breast fed and tries to reproduce them later by thumb-sucking. It is thus that feelings of satiation, security and being loved are inseparable in the infant's early experience.

It is advisable to comply with a baby's tastes and needs as far as is possible in order to make feeding a pleasurable experience and thus ensure the absence of lasting tensions between mother and child. This is the basis of what is known as free-demand feeding. It is recommended by the Aldriches, a medically qualified married couple in the United States. They opposed primarily the kind of infant feeding having a prematurely educational approach. Free-demand feeding involves giving the infant a large measure of freedom in choosing his mealtimes during the first months of life. When the baby is hungry and cries it should immediately be breast fed or given the bottle. The child should also determine the quantity of food; no attempt should be made to force food on him, and it should be withheld only on the doctor's instructions.

The child should never be woken up to be fed. Washing should then be carried out when the child is satisfied and, more often than not, sleepy after being fed. Children fed in this manner fall of their own accord into a rhythm of dozing and sleeping as has been observed among primitive peoples.

In the fourth month the child can be made to wait a short while. He plays by himself, listens and watches, and this is the safest and most suitable time to adapt him to a time schedule.

The opponents of this method stress in particular that the strain on the mother would be unbearable if she had to listen for her child's every cry and be completely at his beck and call. She would become a slave to her child and find it impossible to take into account her own interests or those of other members of the family. The sheer physical and mental strain on the young mother would become a burden and be of no benefit to the newborn baby.

The weakness of this argument is that – as previously stated – children fed on demand fall into their own sleep-wake rhythm, thus enabling the mother to obtain necessary rest. Another point that the opponents of free-demand feeding overlook is that unfulfilled wishes on the part of the child for the food and protection afforded by the mother lead to discomfort that may find expression in paroxysmal weeping, tantrums, sleep disturbances, unrest and digestive disturbances. Infants, whose elementary needs for food and the maternal care accompanying it have been too early frustrated, will in the end make more demands on the mother's attention than those whose cries received timely response and satisfaction.

There is also the danger of lasting developmental disturbances occurring in infants whose vital needs were prematurely thwarted in a manner they cannot possibly grasp at such an early age. When such children are fed they tend to drink hastily and desire large quantities, being seemingly never satisfied. This behavioural pattern is the infant's answer to an insecure and disturbed mother–child relationship. It has been put forward that in such a situation the seeds are sown for later tendencies towards greed, envy and jealousy.

As Freud pointed out, the mother–child relationship is even more important than the method of feeding. Such factors as insufficient love and attention, absentmindedness and hasty or rushed feeding give rise to the first feeling of aggression towards the mother, which the child can neither express nor overcome but only repress. This evokes ambivalent attitudes to the mother. Such conflicting emotions cause various autonomic reactions. On the one hand, the child's body is in a state of readiness for food, on the other, the mother is unconsciously rejected. The sequelae are counter-innervation, stomach cramps and vomiting, which can be the first psychosomatic manifestation of a later neurotic development.

'Three-month colic' is another example we could mention. Insecure, anxious mothers transfer their concern to their child. The insecurity produces increased tension in the infant, together with colicky pains and sudden bouts of crying. The mother thinks her child is hungry, gives it food and thereby increases the tension already present, which again produces colic.

Investigations carried out by Spitz (1945/46) provided striking evidence that adequate feeding of infants, strictly adhering to hygienic principles, but given without manifest loving care fell short of the mark. He made a study of infants brought up in a home where the shortage of nurses resulted in a lack of love and attention, although everything needed from the hygienic and biological points of view was regularly and adequately supplied. A quarter of the children who remained in this situation for more than five months died of nutritional diseases. The remainder exhibited severe mental and physical damage which in a large number of cases remained in evidence for many years. Spitz made the interesting discovery that if the number of nurses was increased so that each child could be picked up while being fed from the bottle, and if the nurses smiled at the children, such disturbances did not occur and those already present disappeared again providing they had not been in existence for longer than five months.

Hufeland had made a similar observation as early as 1798. In his book *Die Künste, das menschliche Leben zu verlängern* (The Art of Prolonging Human Life) he wrote that out of the 7,000 children who were brought to the Foundlings Home in Paris each year only 180 were still alive ten years later. He recognized that the reason for this high mortality rate lay partly in the separation of the children from their mothers and the loveless treatment they received in the home.

Anxious parents often complain to their doctor that their child 'doesn't eat anything'. To such parents the 'care' of the child does not go beyond seeing that he eats enough and empties his bowels regularly. In return they expect rosy cheeks. Coercion and appeals to reason or volition tend to dull the appetite rather than sharpen it. Such children, who really feel neglected and lonely, tend to regard the parents' persuasions as merely a means of achieving their own peace of mind and experience them as subliminal threats of further withdrawal of affection. Children react in extremely varied ways to such parental blackmail. They may eat only when told to do so and then only piecemeal, refuse food in defiance or passively tolerate over-feeding to the point of becoming obese. Effective treatment is only possible once the disturbed relationship underlying the nutritional disorder has been revealed.

Nutrition as a Communicative Experience

We have seen that infant feeding is not merely a matter of metabolism but that it is inseparably linked with feelings of security, of being loved and cared for, or with feelings of a totally opposed kind. Such experience in early life is never completely effaced. Goethe aptly stated in his *Wilhelm Meister* that no-one could escape from the first impressions of his childhood. Symbolic hunger for security, love or recognition can influence the stomach in such a manner that one may experience a longing for food that appears very real. Such hunger frequently results in overeating to the point of phagomania. In his investigations into the etiology of obesity Cremerius (1968) found that this association of symbols was a deciding factor.

Mitscherlich (1961/62) has stated that the tea-breaks taken in offices and other places of work are not really for the purpose of satisfying a calorie need but rather for relieving the listlessness connected with the given situation, just as the infant related the experience of feeding to relief from discomfort.

Eating is indeed eminently suited to reviving moods and feelings experienced in the past and in a similar setting. As excellent an observer as Proust analysed his own feelings on enjoying a cup of tea and a biscuit. In *A la recherche du temps perdu* he wrote: ‘I lifted the spoon to my lips having previously put a piece of biscuit into my mouth. The instant the liquid and the biscuit touched my palate I trembled with the extraordinary sensation that overcame me. As if out of the blue a feeling of enchanting bliss took hold of me, and I was completely unaware of its origin.’

Proust’s previous feeling of wretchedness had disappeared and he wondered from where his new happiness had come. He concentrated on searching for its origin and finally he saw once more a happy picture from his early youth: a Sunday morning when his aunt had brought him tea and biscuits. Everything was there again – the summer house, the neighbour’s garden and Combray; the delightful picture unfolded before his eyes like a Japanese paper flower in a glass of water.

Owing to the close connection between food and mood, mealtimes are the most unsuitable occasions for arguments, correcting children or giving them severe lectures. The annoyance not only ruins the appetite but impedes the process of revitalization that should accompany every meal.

Healthy eating involves more than just healthy food; a friendly atmosphere at the table and food that we like are equally important.

An experiment carried out at the Bethesda Institute near Washington, DC, to test certain psychic influences on appetite and digestibility proved extremely revealing. Several men who were accustomed to plenty of good food volunteered to take part in the experiment. They were given meals consisting of anything they wanted but had to eat the food in pulp form through a tube in a small bare room. The experiment soon had to be abandoned since all the volunteers lost their usual appetite, found the meals disagreable and lost a considerable amount of weight.

An experiment of this type naturally reflects extremes. Nevertheless, for everyday purposes it can be concluded that the way meals are presented and the external circumstances that determine our mealtimes are matters of no mean importance. An attractively laid table and food served in an appetizing way do more than merely satisfy our aesthetic sensibilities. When heightened rather than diminished by outward appearances, the enjoyment of food is also beneficial to health. Because eating is associated in our subconscious with the need for care and affection, loveless 'feeding' signifies a disappointment which if continually repeated can damage our health.

It is not generally known that our psychological needs are reflected in our eating habits. In a fundamental study Kaufmann classified foods according to their psychological implications; positive foods include those with 'safety components' that produce a feeling of security, such as milk, foods that signify thanks or a reward (sweets), foods with a magical action that give strength (beefsteak, black pudding), foods that reflect social standing (caviar and other delicacies), 'adult' refreshments that are forbidden to children (coffee, beer, wine), etc.

Accordingly, the craving for sweetmeats frequently constitutes a form of self-reward when there is a background of boredom and lack of love. Müller-Eckhard aptly commented that many women seek the sweetness at the confectioners that they miss in their love life.

Practical Conclusions

Eating is not only closely related to the need for affectionate attention; indeed, it is even more of a communicative event. Such expression becomes immediately clear when we consider that meals frequently require the work of other people. Moreover, most of us prefer to eat in company with others. A doctor has to take this into consideration when he requests the patient to give up some of his eating habits, which may be one of the few pleasures in his life. A person who has to cut down on his meals or follow a particular diet often feels 'reduced' and deprived of a full life. Without psychological help, therefore, even the right diet could have an unfavourable effect.

For this reason it is essential to give the patient a thorough explanation as to why he is being asked to make such sacrifices. The best results are obtained by arousing the patient's enthusiasm for the desired objective. In prescribing a diet, the doctor must of course consider the patient's financial situation and occupation. Instructions should be precise and easy to understand. Experience has shown that they are most effective when written, provided with the name of the patient, and contain remarks tailored to his individual needs.

It is moreover always advisable to enquire into the eating habits of patients presenting with alimentary disturbances or gastrointestinal disorders. They can provide invaluable clues as to the origin of the patient's abdominal discomfort, loss of appetite or bulimia.

2.3.2 Overnutrition and Obesity

Basic Aspects

Despite all questions that are still open on the problem of obesity, it is at least generally agreed that a positive energy balance lies at the root of the trouble. The food intake of obese patients is more than they actually need. However, they also appear to have a lower basal metabolic rate and are able to keep their weight constant with less food intake than persons of normal weight. This is said to be accompanied by a predominance of parasympathetic innervation and consequent reduction of metabolic processes.

In the overweight, there is a disturbance of the normal satiety control. Pudel (1967) is of the opinion that obese patients are influenced more by external stimuli in their craving for food than they are by physiological internal stimuli. Such patients just do not know when they are hungry. Instead, their appetite is triggered by external stimuli and various forms of discomfort and uneasiness.

The perpetual desire to eat or sudden bulimia are thus not an expression of an increased need for food on the part of the organism. It is rather that when confronted by conflicts and personal problems these patients regress to infantile patterns in attempting to overcome their feelings of discomfort and displeasure. Food then becomes a consolation for satisfying other, unfulfilled emotional needs.

Adiposity and anorexia have a common tangent in the sense that in both there is a dependence on the satisfaction of oral needs. In the former, the fixation is expressed in the form of positive dependence as compulsive overeating, and in the latter in that of negative dependence as a refusal to eat.

Freyberger and Struwe (1962/63) classify the obese according to eating habits into four main groups:

1. The binge-eater. He is suddenly overcome by a voracious appetite. His ecstatic craving becomes uncontrollable and he consumes enormous quantities of food before he is finally satisfied. One even speaks of an 'oral orgasm'.
2. The continual eater. Appetite occurs on getting up in the morning and persists throughout the day. This type of patient can and will eat at any time, being incapable of limiting himself to the main meals of the day. Yet he does not appear to suffer from his compulsion; on the contrary, he feels quite well.
3. The insatiable. Unlike his fellow sufferers in the other groups, appetite does not drive him to a well-laid table. But once he starts to eat, his hunger knows no bounds.

4. The night-eater. This type of patient is most common in the United States and is afflicted by hunger only after nightfall. No matter how much he eats, his hunger remains unsatisfied. His sleep is troubled or he frequently awakes and eats, then goes to bed again and suffers from reduced appetite on the following morning. From this shift in the polarity between hunger and satisfaction, Freyberger concludes that there is a defect in the structure or function of the ventromedial nucleus. But this has so far not been proved.

Personality Profile

Bruch (1957) showed how obesity can be triggered by parents if they respond systematically to the child's every need by offering him something to eat and make their attention dependent on his acceptance. Such behavioural patterns lead to lack of ego strength, so that frustrations can neither be coped with nor worked through but must be compensated by 'reinforcement'. A strong mother fixation is frequently encountered in obese patients. Petzold and Reindell (1980) point out the maternal dominance in such families and the subordinate role played by the father. Bräutigam (1976) describes how these mothers impair the child's motor development and social ability by their excessive care, and fixate him in a passive-receptive attitude.

From the psychosomatic point of view the excessive caloric intake may be explained as a form of defence against emotional tensions, dissatisfactions and anxiety states, particularly those having a depressive undertone. Many members of the lay public are quite aware that excessive weight gain may result from overeating caused by worry.

Yet it is impossible to describe a standard type of obese patient. We encounter traits of inner compulsion, apathetic, gloomy resignation and signs of a flight into isolation. The act of eating shifts the unpleasant affects – even if only briefly – into a depression-free phase.

The patients feel incomplete, vulnerable and inadequate. Hyperphagia, reduced activity and the resultant excess weight provide a certain amount of protection against this deep-seated sense of inadequacy: being large and imposing makes the obese person feel stronger and safer. In isolated cases the bulimia either appears or is reinforced as an obvious result of frustration.

Regressing to the infantile pattern of equating food with love, the obese person often seeks consolation in eating for the affection he lacks.

Treatment

Slimming cures are usually ineffective unless it is possible to change the patient's instinctual-affective behaviour in such a way that he no longer feels that he has to overeat and so become overweight.

On the whole, the results of treatment in general practice have been bad because the pleasure–pain balance is ignored. It is thus repeatedly pointed out that during dieting over half the patients exhibit symptoms of nervousness, irritability, fatigue and depression in the broader sense. All of these may find expression in the patient's increased anxiety.

Reasons for the frequent failure in the treatment of obesity are as follows:

1. In both diagnosis and treatment, the organic approach to medicine tends to concentrate on alterations in physical structures and their functions. The problem of the obese patient has no place in such a concept. In a moral sense he is frequently regarded as being 'foolish' rather than 'ill', the inference being that he himself is responsible for his condition. Emotionally, he is frequently rejected.
2. Careful analysis of the particular behavioural pattern along with its implications and motivations is indispensable for treating a disorder of this kind. For such an undertaking, the doctor frequently has neither adequate training nor time enough at his disposal. It is moreover difficult to offer the patient satisfactory compensation for the loss of pleasure he obtains in eating.
3. Sociological factors also play an important role in epidemiological consideration. We are thinking here of the stimulus and temptation offered by the display and availability of traditional high-calorie foods, against which our treatment is largely powerless.
4. Patients deviate far more frequently from their doctor's instructions than one would like to believe. Such behaviour is a particular source of annoyance to the doctor since he assumes that a patient who does not follow his instructions is not prepared to cooperate. Many investigations have however shown that patients often fail to understand or remember the instructions because they are too complicated. They are also extremely reluctant to ask the doctor to explain or repeat his instructions.

How can patient compliance be motivated? Most important is the patient's *active* participation in the treatment. In order to do this the doctor must first of all establish a good contact with the patient. The better this sympathetic understanding develops, the easier will be his task. Of prime importance is it to form a picture of how deeply the patient is affected in his personality by being deprived of a means of overcoming his conflicts and of obtaining pleasure.

The next step is to draw up an individual plan for treatment together with the patient, taking into account his personal situation and occupation. The reader is here referred to the remarks in the *practical conclusions* in the section on *Nutrition* (page 50). The patient should be offered the possibility of practising and controlling what is for him an unfamiliar eating behaviour. How extremely important this is has been shown in a study carried out by Balabanski and Tashev (1976) according to which, patients who had lost 17 kg could only keep their weight normal if they were given regular weekly consultations by their doctor. Follow-up studies on a group of patients who had broken off contact with their doctor after treatment showed that they had very quickly put on weight again. The application of behaviour therapy techniques and specifically orientated group therapy may also be of help to such patients. Treatment employing exclusively appetite suppressants has, on the other hand, proved of little value.

2.3.3 Anorexia Nervosa

Basic Aspects

The prime characteristic of anorexia nervosa is a radical refusal to eat, causing patients to lose 20–40% of what their weight was at the onset of the disorder. Food intake is reduced so drastically that it is not uncommon for the life of the patient to be endangered. The case fatality rate is about 10%. Women are mostly affected, and in addition to weight loss, the clinical picture is frequently characterized by amenorrhea, usually secondary. Other symptoms are vomiting, constipation, and serious abuse of laxatives and diuretics; another typical feature is energy conservation by vagal inhibition, which is accompanied by hypotension, bradycardia and reduced cardiac output (Deter et al.).

In severe cases the somatic picture is completed by hypoproteinemia, electrolyte shifts and the formation of edema. The psychic pattern of symptoms is characterized by a conspicuous discrepancy between the cachetic state of the body and the psychomotor hyperactivity of these patients, who often participate in sports despite their greatly impaired general condition. In addition to disturbed eating habits, Bruch, and Slade and Russel pointed out the distorted body image of patients with anorexia nervosa. They overestimate, for example, the breadth of their own body considerably. Another striking feature is a disturbed ability to establish human contact, which makes the patients appear affected, cold, and distant. This is complemented by their denial of the condition, which they stubbornly claim to be 'normal' and appear to be proud of any further weight loss. A marked performance orientation and strong control over impulses finally mean that the patients try to concentrate their entire energy on achieving weight losing objectives; control and mastery of their body represents but one further facet of performance they feel they must fulfil to the utmost.

The historical development of this disease concept can be divided into four periods. The first of these covers the early attempts to relate the disorder to some kind of suggestive process. During the second period the symptoms and pathogenesis of the syndrome were more clearly defined. The third phase began in 1914 with Simmonds' discovery of hypophyseal cachexia and the fourth is distinguished by psychoanalytical and phenomenological investigations.

The first paper on anorexia nervosa was published by Porta, a Neapolitan physician practising in the sixteenth century. His monograph bore the title *Reflections of the prominent philosopher Simone Porta of Naples on the case of the young daughter della Magna who lived for two years without eating or drinking* and was translated into the Florentine language by Giovanbattista Galli.

In 1689, in his treatise on phthisis, the English physician Richard Morton described, under the heading 'atrophy or nervous consumption', a loss of body tissue which occurs in the absence of fever, cough or dyspnea but which is accompanied by loss of appetite and marked disturbances of the digestive tract such as achylia and dyspepsia. In Paris in 1873, Lasègue published a fundamental study of anorexia hysterica in which he attributed the disorder to a particular state of mind, in other words to a mental perversion due to the admitted or hidden emotions of the patients.

In the same year William Gull, a Londoner, called the syndrome apepsia hysterica, believing that it was caused by functional impairment of the gastric branches of the vagus nerve in patients with a hysterical disposition. He later used the expression anorexia nervosa.

Owing to Simmonds' description in 1914 of a case of cachexia involving atrophy of the anterior lobe of the pituitary gland, a connection was for many years thought to exist between hypophyseal cachexia and anorexia nervosa, with the result that the latter was treated with pituitary extracts or transplants.

In recent years, however, anorexia nervosa has become more a problem for psychiatrists, who have turned their attention to a phenomenological understanding and interpretation of the disorder (Binswanger 1957; Kuhn 1951, 1953; Kielholz 1966; Keeler quoting Ringel 1969). Zutt has put forward that a cardinal symptom of anorexia is the inability of the patients to eat together with others. This he regards as a communicative disorder underlying the disturbed eating pattern.

Personality Profile

The patient usually comes from a middle-class family and is often the only daughter. If she has brothers, she almost invariably complains of being regarded as inferior to them (Jores 1976). Most patients give the impression of being well-adapted, conscientious, and obedient to the point of docility. They are usually of high intelligence and make brilliant scholars. Their interests are centred around intellectual subjects, their ideals ascetic. They are usually good at their work and have a high degree of general competence.

The situation triggering the disturbed eating behaviour is not uncommonly the first erotic experience, which the patients cannot work through, and find threatening. Other precipitating factors may be intense rivalry with their brothers and sisters, separation anxiety by the death of grandparents, divorce, or grown-up children leaving the family circle.

At the centre of the psychodynamic pattern of forces is a symbiotic bondage to the mother coupled with a strong, ambivalent desire to distance herself (Ziolko 1985). On the one hand, the patients turn their self-destroying aggression against themselves as punishment for their 'betrayal' in desiring to be separated from the mother. On the other, they attempt to use their rejection of food in order to gain loving care or, if this fails, at least to annoy the other members of the family, particularly the mother, and exercise control over them (Schaefer and Martin quoting Schaefer and Schwarz 1974). In many of these families, the dominant topic giving rise to vexatious reactions is in fact the patient's eating behaviour. When under treatment, the patients attempt to transfer this scheme of reference to the hospital staff.

The same ambivalence becomes apparent if the refusal to eat is regarded as an oral protest. This is primarily directed against the mother, who is not really nurturing the child and yet is not prepared to give her the freedom she requires. The purpose of the protest is equally ambivalent: on the one hand it is an attempt to extort affectionate care, while on the other, food is rejected in an effort to gain independence. It is precisely this striving for self-sufficiency that paradoxically leads to self-destruction when taken to its logical conclusion.

In anorexia nervosa it is thus not simply oral aggression that is suppressed – the negation relates to all oral needs and the ego attempts to assert itself and gain importance by rejecting all oral stimuli. In this disorder it seems that the idea of 'having to lose weight' constitutes from the onset an immutable component of the personality. The peculiarity is found only in symptoms triggered by psychotic processes. Even in severe forms of anorexia, the ego does not fight against the idea by which it is dominated; this also explains the lack of awareness of the disorder and the refusal of all help.

Selvini-Palazzoli et al. (1977; Selvini-Palazzoli 1975) accordingly speak of a monosymptomatic psychosis restricted to the dominating idea that the body must be destroyed by the denial of all oral tendencies. Clauser (1976) described anorexia nervosa as a chronic form of suicide.

The psychodynamic interpretation is thus: the patients transfer their struggle against instinctual drives, particularly those of a sexual nature, to an oral plane by refusing to eat. Anorexia nervosa has also been interpreted as a flight from womanhood, and it must be admitted that the desired results are achieved in that the development of the characteristically feminine form is halted. It is interesting to note that many patients state the reason for their behaviour as the wish to "avoid at any price getting a fat belly". Looked at in this way, the refusal to eat may also represent a defence against vague fears of pregnancy.

The rejection of food does not however constitute solely a struggle against the maturing of feminine sexuality. It is an attempt to resist becoming adult, backed by a feeling of helplessness at the thought of the increasing demands imposed by the process.

However, not only the patient's own psychodynamic profile is important in making a diagnosis and prescribing treatment; there has been a tendency in recent years to devote more attention to the interplay of relationships in the patient's family. The general attitude of life prevailing in this unit is often orientated towards perfectionism, ambition, and achievement. Interaction between its members is strongly determined by watchful, over-attentive, and harmonizing impulses. Emotional conflicts are stubbornly disclaimed since none of the family see any possibility of working out adequate solutions for them. The atmosphere in the home is therefore constantly tense though outwardly it may present a solid picture of concord and harmony.

Minuchin (1977; Minuchin et al. 1983) listed the behavioural characteristics of these families: complex involvement, over-attentiveness, avoidance of conflict, stubbornness, and children implicated in parents' quarrels. For him the symptoms of anorexia nervosa constitute a power struggle of the daughter versus her parents within the context of a grossly entangled relationship in which the patient's body constitutes 'the last ditch' in retaining some degree of autonomy in the face of parents' demands.

Selvini-Palazzoli et al. observed that each member of the family seems concerned with forcing his own definition of the relationship on another. Conversely, each rejects .the other's definition. No one is prepared to assume leadership openly and accept responsibility for decisions. Overt alliances between two members of the family are unthinkable. 'Coalitions' across the age-gap are disclaimed at verbal levels even when otherwise obvious. Behind the facade of married accord and harmony lurks a deep mutual disenchantment that will, however, never be admitted.

In an attempt to shed more light on the symptoms within a familial context, Selvini-Palazzoli commented:

> In a system where every attempt at communication will most likely meet with refusal, the refusal to eat would seem to be in complete accord with the family style of interaction. It conforms particularly to the group's expiatory frame of mind, in which suffering appears to be the winning move.

The patient's family is generally dominated by a female authority figure, which may be the mother or a grandmother. The father is excluded from the child's emotional sphere, being outmanoeuvred and belittled by the mother, either openly or otherwise. The father generally responds by retreating further from the scene, with the result that the mother thinks she must consolidate and extend her position of dominance.

Wirsching and Stierlin describe the characteristic features of families with an anorectic daughter as being exaggerated expectations of achievement on the part of the parents, a family ideal of selflessness with corresponding competition among its members.

Treatment

The general practitioner's first duty is to make sure there is no organic cause for the disorder. When making a differential diagnosis particular attention should be paid to wasting diseases such as tuberculosis, malignant tumours and hyperthyroidism, and also to chronic enteritis and juvenile diabetes.

A disorder which for many years was often confused with anorexia nervosa is Simmonds' hypophyseal cachexia.

Anorexia nervosa should then be distinguished from symptomatic anorexia occurring in cases of depression or schizophrenia where sitophobia could, for example, be due to fear of poisoning. A finer distinction must also be made between reactive anorexia from psychogenic inhibition and vomiting neurosis due to emotional trauma resulting from mechanical function disorders of the digestive tract and leading to an involuntary weight loss (esophagospasm, functional dysphagia, intractable vomiting, etc.).

Petzold (1979) attaches great importance to general medical care. He sees its primary task as being that of no more but no less than to conserve what remains. A frequent problem is to keep informed about the patient's weight and nutritional state without oppressing her with too many check-ups since the disorder represents in the first place a protest against excessive family control.

Early diagnosis is of prime importance since the prospects of successful treatment diminish as the disease progresses.

The initial contact is rendered difficult by the patients' cool, passive and often mistrustful attitude. Freud refused to give treatment on an outpatient basis. He considered that these patients, who were so near to death, had the ability to gain such a mastery over their analyst that it was impossible for him to overcome their resistance (Freud, quoted from Köhle and Simons 1979).

The patients' lack of insight into their illness makes it particularly difficult for the treatment to take shape. Ziolko (1971) spoke of an 'exchange of blows' with the doctor that can end in the patient's favour by her achieving a minimal weight. Kütemeyer reported that more effort and attention had to be devoted to one patient's problems with other patients, other doctors and the hospital staff in general than to the patient herself. With the passage of time these problems increased in such measure that the growing conflict of opposing impulses gave an impression of whimsicality and extreme malice.

A vast range of therapeutic measures have been suggested by various authors over the past thirty years. The sheer weight of numbers and the frequent contradictions between the individual recommendations are indicative of the uncertainty of the results and the lack of specific remedies.

In recent years there has been an increasing tendency to recommend treatment employing a combined approach carried out by well-coordinated teams in special centres. The initial phase of treatment consists of feeding up the patient. Should behaviour therapy fail to bring about a change for the better, the nasogastric tube must be resorted to in order to avert the progressive threat to the patient's life. Feeding by intubation is then replaced at a later phase by measures involving behaviour therapy. The treatment is based on the principle of operant conditioning. The patients are isolated but the situation is improved by the presence of the therapist at mealtimes. During the initial stages of treatment the patient is rewarded for every increase in weight, while at a later stage the reward is given for maintaining what is considered as a normal weight.

The problem for the doctor handling such cases is to avoid giving the impression of forcing the patient to eat or allowing the symptoms of the disease to become the focal topic of the treatment. Indeed, the aim is to break any tendency on the part of the patient to restrict her perceptions to purely physiological aspects.

In addition to behaviour therapy, various forms of treatment incorporating depth psychology and body therapies have been employed with varying degrees of success. Most authors now agree that inclusion of the patient's family in the main therapeutic setting produces better results than individual therapy. Moreover, when family perspectives are also given consideration, inpatient treatment appears to be more successful than outpatient therapy alone (von Rad and Senf; Petzold 1983).

In a follow-up study, Minuchin et al. found that over 80% of the patients were cured. Unfortunately, few centres are in a position to carry out such highly-qualified family therapy. When, however, the psychodynamic aspects of the patient's family are taken into account, the rule of thumb no longer applies that 10% of cases have fatal outcome, that one third remain anorectic, that the disorder becomes chronic and a further third develop severe emotional, even psychotic symptoms after losing those of anorexia nervosa, while only the remainder show a change for the better (Cremerius 1965). With the improved treatment now available, such results may be illustrative but are henceforth outdated.

2.3.4 Bulimia

Basic Aspects

Bulimia ('hunger of an ox') is associated with bulmorexia or over-eating usually followed by induced vomiting. The principal symptoms are

- frequent eating bouts of limited duration,
- active weight control by vomiting or abuse of laxatives.

The eating bouts or binges are not, by definition, attributable to either anorexia nervosa or somatic illness. Bulimia differs from the former in that patients are usually of normal weight and the desire for extreme reducing is absent. However, Ziolko (1985) sees both disorders as polarities of one and the same disease, dysorexia, bulimia being distinguished by fear of weight gain coupled with a craving for food. According to Habermas and Müller, the earliest description of bulimia stems from Wulf in 1932, who described '. . . an interesting complex of oral symptoms and its relation to addiction'.

Women in the 15–25-year age group are affected by this disorder far more than men. The patients come mostly from middle and higher class families. Similar to the situation with anorexia nervosa, it would seem that the clinical picture has intensified in recent years. This may relate to increased publicity and more tendency on the part of patients – whose disorders are frequently chronic – to seek medical aid. Many patients are noticed only after concomitant somatic symptoms have been observed. Abuse of laxatives and diuretics may cause electrolyte imbalance and edema. Esophagitis, dental lesions, and chronic swelling of the parotid gland are sequels to vomiting gastric juices.

Frequent mastication leads to hypertrophy of the masseter muscle, giving patients their characteristic facial appearance. Distension of the stomach, constipation after laxative abuse, and menstrual disorders complete the somatic picture.

Bulimia is sometimes referred to as the secret sister of anorexia since patients may succeed in hiding their symptoms over the years; only after direct questioning do they admit to binges followed by self-induced vomiting and laxative abuse. These are often planned, or form part of a daily ritual. Large amounts, sometimes up to 10,000 kcal, of high energy value food are consumed within a short time. After a brief period of relief, the bouts are followed by vague, inner tensions and severe feelings of shame and guilt.

Personality Profile

The patients give an initial impression of strength, independence, ambition, single-mindedness and even self-control. But their outward image differs greatly from the one they have of themselves – utter emptiness and no sense of purpose. They also indulge in pessimistic or depressive moods resulting from patterns of thought and behaviour that fuel feelings of helplessness, shame, guilt and insufficiency (Habermas and Müller). Self image and self ideal are poles apart, so the patients tend to live the good life in public and a miserable one in private.

They frequently stem from families whose members are likely to act on impulse and where potential violence figures high. Johnson and Flach reported on increased occurrence of affective psychoses in relatives of the first degree: fathers tended to have alcohol problems, mothers were overweight, and food problems became topic number one. The structures of such families tended to be marked by conflict and impulsiveness; few ties existed within the family nucleus; stress was present in abundance and success in solving problems very limited. In this milieu, moreover, there was a high degree of social pressure on achievement.

It is a situation in which the patients assume responsibilities and parental functions at an early age. Sentiments of not getting one's fair share and of being at the mercy of the parents' moods and whims are countered by a kind of behaviour that is full of concern; the helplessness and dependence of the essential individual are held in check till finally vented in alternate bouts of eating and vomiting.

Emotional instability, impulsiveness coupled with the fear of losing control, low frustration tolerance, and a high degree of addictive potential determine the psychodynamic aspect. The patients do not always succeed in critically perceiving and expressing their intrapsychic state. They thus experience vague feelings of some growing, deep threat about to engulf them.

Since formulation of the conflict is impossible, the defence mechanism of displacement occurs orally, and eating acquires a different significance. Hunger is misinterpreted as a threat, as a loss of bodily control, which is equated with an inability to master life. The binge itself does have stress reducing, integrating functions in the sense of a self-consolatory act. But relief is impermanent, and the patient subsequently experiences the bout as a loss of control radically jeopardizing her autonomy and mastery over life. Vomiting is induced in order to keep bodyweight constant, which the patient considers an indicator of restored self-control and self-determination. Feelings of guilt and shame about what has happened are then often the cause for social and emotional withdrawal as well as for the cleavage of a very presentable external image from a secret one that leaves much to be desired. The discrepancy between the self-concept and social image can provoke feelings of inner emptiness and tension. These in turn may be activated under stressful situations to trigger anew the vicious circle of the illness.

Treatment

Patients are generally unable to limit the strong surge of their symptoms unless these are made the centre of some structuring form of therapy. An attempt should be made to agree on a plan of regular mealtimes, and weight kept constant by not exceeding a certain caloric intake. This may prove helpful when complemented by the following strategy: The patient is encouraged to write down her feelings, thoughts and experiences at the time of the bout or note those that trigger it off. Alternative methods must be kept in view, such as establishing contacts with certain friends or relatives or embarking on different activities.

Since recurrence is frequent, preventive measures to counter disappointment are necessary. These are aimed at relieving the patient of feelings of shame and guilt and avoiding too high expectations.

These methods, possibly reinforced by a self-help group, will, in favourable instances, succeed in releasing the energy at the root of the symptom and rechannel it to develop innate creative potential. In the majority of cases, however, more advanced psychotherapeutic measures are needed. These are aimed at depriving the symptoms of their ego-alien compulsive character; it is made clear to the patient that as far as the triggering situation is concerned such symptoms are a ‘meaningful’, if unsuccessful, attempt to solve the conflict, and that more effective means are readily available.

Group and individual therapies are indicated when symptomatic treatment alone does not give adequate relief. Habermas and Müller point out, however, that individual therapy tends to create a situation marked by the all-or-none way of thinking and strong idealization of the therapist. This attitude towards the therapist can suffer total reversal at the first hint of disappointment ('whoever doesn't understand me fully doesn't understand me at all!' 'One mistake and all is lost!').

In severe cases the structuring needed can be ensured only by treatment under hospitalization.

As in the treatment of anorexia nervosa, family therapy gives positive results. It has still not been shown whether it is superior to either individual or group therapies. Owing to the high potential of familial conflict, no treatment can afford to neglect such psychodynamic aspects.

2.4 Gastrointestinal Disorders

Psychosomatic research has shown that the emotions playing a significant role in the development of gastrointestinal and nutritional disorders are quite specific in their nature. They are mostly centred around a yearning for security and protection. In order to achieve this, most of the patients adopt a regressive course, following a rather infantile pattern of behaviour.

It is hardly surprising that security has gained such a position of precedence in our present day and age. The hazards to which civilized man is exposed have an increasing tendency to exceed all accustomed dimensions and assume a more anonymous character. Moreover, it is particularly the more advanced countries that are in the throes of restructuring processes. These are rapidly dissolving the protective patriarchal system of order in many domains, particularly in those of the family and religious institutions. Thus at the very time that people are especially conscious of the dangers threatening them, they are confronted with the problem of assuming full responsibility themselves. Many are incapable of coping with these demands and resort to regressive defence mechanisms under stress situations.

Not only eating behaviour but the digestive system too is extremely suited to reflecting somatically problems of security and protection; food represents the primal form of possession for ensuring existence, and digestion the earliest of all forms of 'managing' and utilizing something acquired.

With the development of the human personality, the maturing of emotional and physical qualities, and the emergence of conscience, these basic tendencies evolve in a most complex manner: atonement may be expressed by a refusal to eat, guilt or defiance by vomiting. Bulimia becomes a symptom of a regressive striving for security in the face of excessive demands.

Greed and aspirations for power may go hand in hand with endeavours to gain security and acquire possessions; events associated with intestinal contents reflect problems involved in giving and retaining, as well as in ambition and obsessive obedience on the one hand and defiance and dependence on the other.

With regard to their pronounced regressive features, gastrointestinal disorders have something in common with addiction and depression, which have shown such a marked increase in recent years. Unlike these disorders, however, the background of emotional events in gastrointestinal illness is more masked than exhibited: only the physical symptom remains apparent. If the target symptom or organ is eventually cured by medical or surgical means (stomach ulcer, ulcerative colitis), psychic symptoms such as anxiety, depression or addiction frequently become manifest.

From the point of view of existential analysis, however, physical symptoms are understood in the context of the basic mental make-up. Using this phenomenological approach, Staehelin (1963) sees gastrointestinal symptoms as the expression of the following emotional factors:

difficulty in grasping hold of things (stomatitis, gingival disorders);
difficulty in 'swallowing' something (eating and deglutition disorders);
feelings of disgust or repulsion (anorexia, nausea, vomiting, emaciation);
chronic 'mental indigestion', difficulty in mastering something (gastralgia, hypermotility, pylorospasm, ulcer);
chronic inability to work something through (pain, enterocolitis, irritable colon);
inability to part with something (chronic constipation);
desire to get rid of something (chronic diarrhea).

2.4.1 Gastric and Duodenal Ulcers

Basic Aspects
Glatzel described peptic ulceration as the development of gastric and duodenal ulcers arising in certain stressful situations in persons predisposed to react to such experience with somatic disorders of the gastrointestinal tract by virtue of their personality structure and life history.

He distinguished ulcers produced in this manner from those due to purely physical causes such as burns, poisoning, infections and circulatory disturbances. Duodenal ulcers occur exclusively in patients having a tendency to hypersecretion – frequently from birth.

Gastric functions, motoricity, blood flow and secretion are closely connected with the activity of superposed nervous processes as well as with the prevailing emotional state. Aggressiveness and resentment accelerate the passage of food through the stomach, whereas anxiety and strong emotions cause pylorospasm and slow it down. Anxiety, an unrealizable desire to flee, depressive thoughts or low spirits reduce hydrochloric acid secretion, motility and blood flow in the stomach. Chronic anxiety and conflict states that produce hostile reactions and aggressive tendencies increase gastric secretion and, if they persist, cause mucosal changes such as occur in gastritis. A mucosa that has undergone changes in this way seems to be particularly vulnerable to damage: a slight trauma can cause a very small erosion which, through constant contact with the gastric juices, may lead to ulcer formation.

The symptoms are described by patients in many different ways, from 'low gurgling noises' to 'gnawing pains' and an empty feeling in the morning. Some refer to the sensation of internal vibrations and trembling and even a burning feeling in the chest. One patient said he felt as if a flower was opening inside him and something very unpleasant would come out. Only the heart rivals the abdominal region in such high 'anxiety potential'. Both real and feigned functional disturbances may produce feelings of anxiety. Such elements of anxiety influence in turn the nervous system, giving rise to spasm and tension, which complete the vicious circle of symptoms.

The numerous investigations into the causes of peptic ulceration have yielded very different opinions. We reproduce here that of Alexander, firstly because it represents the first description (1934) of the 'psychosomatic structure' of an ulcer patient and secondly because it can be taken as a model for a general approach to psychosomatic disorders in that it attempts to correlate physiological findings with the psychoanalytical theory of neurosis.

Alexander states that ulcer patients do not fall into any characteristic personality group. However, there is always a conflict situation, in which desires and needs arising from the oral sphere of experience (affection, reward, and dependence) are thwarted. This frustration is transformed by a regressive mechanism into a need to be given food. As a result, the stomach receives vagal stimuli even outside of the digestion phase.

Personality Profile

Overbeck and Biebl have suggested the following classification of ulcer personalities, which is not orientated exclusively towards the psychoanalytical model of neurosis:

1. *Emotionally 'Healthy' Patients*. Their personalities possess good ego functions and stable object relationships. They acquire ulcers as a singly occurring psychosomatic reaction to extreme stress of a psychosocial character, which may be specific or nonspecific but originates from the oral sphere of experience. This is accompanied by strong ego regression and resomatization, and, given a certain gastric disposition, ulcer formation occurs. (This is not peptic ulceration in the narrow sense of the word.)
2. *Patients with Character Neurosis*. These patients are prone to pseudo-independent reaction formations or have compulsive-depressive traits. Oral conflicts are apparent to others of their milieu. An example would be the

'executive type' who tends to disseminate aggressive tension. The conflicts eventually enter into a chronic phase under special circumstances such as illness, failure or loss of a love object. They then decompensate with ulcer formation after secondary repression.

3. *Tyrannical Patients*. The characteristics of this group are ego weakness, passive dependence and extreme object dependence. Such patients have a tendency towards impulsive outbursts or litigious paranoiac modes of behaviour. They also act out their oral conflicts as asocial patients (alcoholism, pension neurosis). They fall ill at the faintest suggestion of failure in the sphere of affection and attention. Their gastrointestinal disorder would appear understandable as a physical expression or physiological correlate of their emotional needs.

4. *'Psychosomatic' Ulcer Patients*. Their personalities lack expressive and imaginative faculties. Such patients have a peculiarly rigid, pedestrian way of life and object relationship, which present an impression of complete vacuity to the examining doctor. They appear, moreover, capable only of seeing themselves in other people, and habitually react psychosomatically to any stress or crisis – which is, however, frequently connected with object loss. Their peptic ulceration is often accompanied by other psychosomatic disorders such as febrile reactions, cardiac symptoms, rheumatism, tuberculosis, etc. Furthermore, these patients have usually had a whole series of accidents and operations.

5. *'Normopathic' Patients*. The final group comprises patients who are extremely concerned with exhibiting normal behaviour. They are overadapted, their ego being restricted owing to strong denial strategies (with respect to reality, their own state of exhaustion and physical condition). They are mostly manual or clerical workers, frequently carrying out two occupations, who are involved in a self-destructive, stressful course of action from which they fall victim to a precipitate pattern of ulcerative symptoms.

Much attention has been devoted to the passive and hyperactive types of duodenal ulcer patients in psychosomatic literature. The basic mood of the passive type of patient is rather depressive, and dependency needs are expressed in a direct manner. According to Freyberger (1972), the ulcerations occur when unconscious or conscious desires connected with this dependency suffer a setback.

Of prime importance in the passive type of ulcer patient is an unconscious fear of losing the care and protection afforded by the mother. It is a fear that leads to constant tension. These individuals seek people who are just not *capable* of deserting them and the situation from which they cannot escape. There are those who are not *capable* of believing that their wife no longer loves them. Every doubt, such as the absence of an affectionate regard, may precipitate anxiety. The same reaction may however be produced by fear of an authoritarian father figure. No steps are taken in order to achieve independence. They savour their dependence without assuming any risk themselves. Their whole life strategy is centred on being protected. Balint termed them the dependent 'ocnophiles' as opposed to the venturesome 'philobates'.

These overtly dependent, passive type of ulcer patients mostly originate from overorganized families, in which they were spoiled by a very attentive mother. They have not been able to sever or wean themselves in the psychological sense from their mother. In their desire for help and protection they remain strongly attached to the mother figure, while the father can assume merely a commendatory attitude. W. Loch describes the incapacity of certain patients of proving themselves as good a man as their father and receiving the approval of other men.

These patients also allow themselves to be guided by their need for loving care in their choice of partner. The males of this type of ulcer patient often seek out a mother figure as wife.

Although the dependency needs of '*hyperactive*' *ulcer patients* are also pronounced, they are resisted. These patients attempt to subdue their desire to gratify oral impulses and continue to be frustrated.

According to Alexander, the conflict of this type of ulcer patient is that strong oral-receptive tendencies are rejected because they are incompatible with the strivings of the ego for independence and action. The conscious attitude of these patients may be expressed as follows: I am active and industrious; I like giving things to other people, helping them, assuming responsibility, being a leader; I am an active, even aggressive person who enjoys being left to his own devices. Yet on investigation we find exactly the opposite attitude in his unconscious: a strong yearning for affection and a need for someone to lean on.

The hyperactive type is never at peace with himself. He pursues aggressively his objective by a compensatory striving for independence and a continual, compulsive urge to 'prove himself'. The patient is in need of such confirmation since, for him, success is the only security. Yet the very success he seeks eludes him because the aim of his aspirations is really to win affectionate admiration and prestige. These are the Don Juans in the realm of achievement, active yet uncertain.

In a large-scale trial, Weiner et al. and Mirsky investigated whether it was possible to predict on the basis of psychological criteria which subjects with a tendency to hypersecretion would develop duodenal ulcers.

From 2,073 army conscripts they selected 63 having particularly high amounts of pepsinogen (hypersectetion) and 57 with very low amounts (hyposecretion). The psychological criteria used in forecasting were needs for dependence and attention, which in all likelihood would be frustrated during primary training. On the basis of these criteria it was predicted that 10 of the 120 men chosen had high chances of developing duodenal ulcers.

Of those seen as being particularly susceptible to the illness, 7 were later proved by radiography to have developed duodenal ulcers. Among the 3 who did not have ulcers was 1 from the group having hyposecretion. 2

others of the total group of 120 subjects (both with hypersecretion) were also shown to have developed duodenal ulcers.

Of the 120 recruits examined, 9 can thus be said to have developed duodenal ulcers, all of whom had hypersecretion. 7 of the 9 patients belonged to the 8% classified as being particularly endangered.

The foundation has thus been laid for a hypothetical model of duodenal ulcer formation, in which the central emotional role is played by the patient's dependency needs and desire for care and attention.

Zander is of the opinion, however, that this aspect has so far been ascribed too much importance. He thinks that an unacknowledged envy conflict is responsible for precipitating the disorder. In 70 out of 77 patients Zander found envy of possession and prestige, and only to a lesser extent of interpersonal relationships, to be the triggering factor of duodenal ulcer. Accordingly, an ulcer would develop if someone who felt hungry was obliged to watch others being served with food.

With the assistance of a radiologist 17 patients were placed before the x-ray screen and subjected to an eleven-point interview broaching problems of envy and hunger by posing standard questions. The radiologist recorded his findings on any changes in gastric functions for each of the eleven points.

In the course of the observations, surprising reactions in gastric motility became apparent. During the discussion on the precipitating situation, 15 of the 17 patients showed signs of considerable spasm that increased in intensity towards the pylorus and was identifiable by its characteristic triangular shape. This change in shape usually took place spontaneously, frequently when the only triggering factor mentioned was the *person* involved, and often before the patient's verbal reaction.

According to Deyhle and Jenny the number of patients uprooted from their original surroundings is significantly higher for ulcer patients than for others. In a study on 100 patients with epigastric complaints, they showed that 80% of patients in which duodenal ulcers had been diagnosed had moved to new surroundings. The corresponding figure for patients with other diagnosed disorders was only 35% and 47% for those found normal. This result is important particularly with regard to the frequent sickness found in foreign workers.

Treatment

1. *General Remarks.* With the advent of the H_2-receptor blockers, extremely effective medication is now available. If for no other reason, the considerable pain frequently involved in ulcerative disorders makes medical treatment indispensable. As treatment progresses it can become an important link in doctor–patient relations. In the acute phase, discussions revealing conflicts should be avoided and directed towards effecting changes in the everyday life of the patient. From a psychotherapeutic aspect, attempts to influence somatic functions giving rise to ulcer formation can only be undertaken on a long-term basis. During treatment the doctor should decide

which type of ulcer patient he has; the passive type requires a rather protective doctor–patient relationship and the gentle art of persuasion for taking medicaments as prescribed. The hyperactive ulcer patient requires a different approach: the doctor must insist on his instructions being followed yet keep a weather eye on the patient's conflict of aspirations to independence and needs for dependence.

Autogenic training developed by Schultz has proved of great value in ulcer patients. As is frequently the case in psychosomatic patients, group therapy offers considerable advantages over individual treatment. It is particularly important that the hyperactive patient learns that an active life is also possible in a state of relaxation. A degree of positive transference to the therapist also proves advantageous in this type of treatment.

Particular care should be taken that the patient obtains the help he unconsciously solicits. This demands some reflection on the part of the doctor regarding the meaning of the symptoms and the ability to interpret frequent requests for further examinations, medicaments or an operation (passive attitude) in relation to the patient's life history and situation. Such wishes on the part of the patient should by no means be gratified under coercion.

Paradoxically, it is not infrequent for an ulcer patient to become emotionally stabilized after surgical intervention. One could speak of 'psychosomatics with the knife'. The patient's status as a sick person has then been 'legalized' in the eyes of those around him, and he is regarded and accepted as being 'really ill'. He can finally voice his desire for independence freely without having to fear being branded a failure like so many psychosomatic patients. However, should the emotional problems remain unresolved, quite specific hazards are incurred in surgical treatment, particularly when carried out at an early stage: there may be merely a change in the nature of the symptoms because the dynamics of the unconscious conflict are still effective. According to Freyberger and Leutner, shifts in symptoms occur after operations in the gastric region not infrequently in the form of alcohol abuse, psychoneurotic symptoms, or the latter coupled with psychosomatic or purely somatic symptoms.

2. *Psychotherapeutic Possibilities*. Meyer has pointed out that ulcer patients accept psychotherapy only with reluctance. He explains that 'pseudo-independent' persons resist being dependent on psychotherapists and tend to break off treatment at the first sign of an improvement in their symptoms. Overtly dependent types of patient become disappointed by the prohibitive element present in traditional psychotherapy. Long-term psychotherapy is thus usually unsuitable for ulcer patients.

Modified forms of psychotherapy are however quite applicable, the supportive form being particularly suitable for the passive type of ulcer patients. The patient must be in a position to express his dependency needs without fearing a depreciatory assessment on the part of the doctor. If he has no need to conceal aggressive tendencies owing to a feeling of guilt, he may percieve the doctor as a parental figure and begin to reveal his secret fears. It may thus be possible to verbalize conflicts, discuss problems on a rational level and reduce internal stress.

If the general practitioner or internist prepares himself for this task, say, by attending Balint groups, he will be in a position to apply a form of psychotherapy that meets the main requirements for such cases.

It can hardly be emphasized enough that the effect the discussions have on the patient depends less on the time at the doctor's disposal than on his training in psychosomatic aspects. This alone can improve the ultimate results of treatment by a possible reduction in the number of relapses, a decrease in chronic states and avoidance of surgical procedures.

3. *Family Confrontation*. The effects of the treatment are enhanced when it is possible to include members of the patient's family in the therapeutic procedure. For this purpose, Luban-Plozza has introduced 'family confrontation' into the treatment of psychosomatic patients.

The family forms an integral unit, the sick member of which is the most sensitive and becomes the 'carrier' of familial conflicts. The dynamic approach to emotional forces involved in the family confrontation can effect a considerable saving of time in the treatment administered. The more the family acquires a sense of responsibility in contributing to the therapy and the patient feels he is being understood, the better are the prospects of a cure.

The incorporation of the family into the general therapeutic process is also helpful because ulcer patients are frequently found to have a long family history of similar disorders, in which relationships to the family as a whole, to a marriage partner or to children constitute the source of many different kinds of conflict. Moreover, family confrontation has a prophylactic value in that it helps forestall a certain degree of psychological, hereditary predisposition to ulcer formation; the elimination of misunderstandings and intrafamilial conflict situations can prevent the early problems of interaction so typical of ulcer patients in coming generations.

Further details are contained in Chapter 11 dealing with the rudiments of treatment.

2.4.2 Constipation

Basic Aspects

Most healthy people pass 100–200 g of relatively soft stool daily. One speaks of constipation when several days elapse without any spontaneous bowel movement and the stool is very hard.

Chronic constipation is a frequent and widespread disorder. A large proportion of the female population in particular are dependent on some form of medication in order to achieve bowel movement. About 35% of all women going out to work and 10% of all men have a tendency to constipation, and some 25% of these people take laxatives regularly. Should such complaints be of a protracted nature, it is also quite possible that a somatic cause exists.

Personality Profile
Chronic constipation usually occurs in patients with anxiety and depression who, although outwardly placid, are inwardly tense, deprived of contact and dispirited. Alexander typified their attitude in the sentence: 'I cannot expect anything from anyone else and therefore I don't need to give anything – I must make sure I don't lose what I have.' Freud spoke in this connection of the triad comprising obstinacy, orderliness and thrift, the extremes of which may be intolerance, pedantry and avarice.

Constipation sometimes develops, however, as compensation for a rather voluptuous generosity. In this case, those affected are goodnatured people who tend to give their utmost in every situation, often to the point of exhaustion. Perhaps this explains the stronger predisposition of women to this disorder; the readiness to make sacrifices has always had a major significance in their social evolution.

These patients, whether men or women, are frequently excessively bowel conscious. A 41-year-old civil engineer submitted us a graph on which he had plotted daily the weight of his stool in milligrammes over a period of three months.

Schwidder noted the following correlations with chronic constipation:

1. The body's part in a protest reaction.
2. Attempt at retention, in order to gain mastery or persist.
3. Anxious restraint.
4. Anxiety and defence in the face of overtaxing situations.
5. Defecation is associated with 'dirty' impulses, which are experienced with feelings of guilt or impending danger and are to be guarded against.

Chronic constipation in infancy should generally be regarded as a protest reaction, particularly as a protest against excessive toilet training. Fromm-Reichmann reported on a 3-and-a-half-year-old girl who stubbornly defied her parent's request that she empty her bowels even when she had to sit for prolonged periods on her potty. Yet once she had stood up and dressed, she did it in her panties.

History taking revealed that the father had insisted on an accurate daily report on the child's stool, had shown concern when bowel movement had not taken place and heaped reproaches on the mother. The daughter, however, had been constantly overwhelmed by his pleas and expressions of endearment.

The child analyst soon realized that the anal character components of the father, whose concern for his daughter was identical with his concern for her stool, had begun to produce a child neurosis. By means of her bowel functions, the daughter was able to tyrannize her parents, make them quarrel and gain the attention of her father.

After the parents had taken the doctor's advice not to bother any more about their daughter's stool, this habitually docile child was then obliged to give vent openly to the feelings of defiance and aggression that she had expressed earlier by constipation. When the parents no longer fell for the game with the potty, the child reacted with tantrums. After the first outburst of rage a change set in, marked initially by relapses. After a deaf ear had been turned to the 'bowel language', the child defecated normally and sought new ways of expressing impulses and affects that had formerly been so closely geared to bowel function.

Treatment

Diet and training may have surprisingly good results. Autogenic training too has proved of considerable value in the treatment of chronic constipation. It primarily enables the patient to exercise 'letting himself go' and adopt a more yielding attitude. Should these means prove ineffective, symptom-orientated psychotherapeutic discussions are indicated, which in the long run give good results.

2.4.3 Emotional Diarrhea

This is one of the most frequent functional disturbances of the bowel. It is associated with hypermotility of the large intestine and involves diarrhea alternating with constipation. The disorder may be accompanied by atypical autonomic disturbances. The underlying causes of the bouts are usually situations evidencing anxiety or overstrain, which are in turn bound up with the 'giving up-given up' complex of feelings.

The personality appears to be marked by a fear of authority and a sense of helpless dependence. Impressions of being subjected to excessive demands, together with feelings of weakness, are overcompensated by an exaggerated desire for recognition and achievement.

The anxiety and overstrain chronically experienced by the patient are best illustrated by words describing the momentary fears of the examination candidate or unaccustomed public speaker: 'He sees himself foundering, helpless and overwhelmed. His only hope of gaining recognition is by yielding, giving' (Bräutigam and Christian). His bowel content represents an infantile form of gift.

Medicamentation alone is clearly inadequate for treatment. The underlying conflict can be successfully worked through in the course of individual or group therapy, provided the patient is sufficiently motivated to accept it.

2.4.4 Irritable Colon

Synonyms are spastic colon, spastic constipation, and irritable bowel syndrome. Up to 50% of all patients consulting a doctor on account of abdominal complaints have this symptom complex, which is characterized by diffuse pain, alternating constipation and diarrhea, and frequently by distention in this region (the 'bloated belly'). All symptoms can be worsened by emotional aspects and stress situations.

Differential diagnosis is complicated since it involves excluding all other disorders of the gastrointestinal tract.

Petzel and Reindell (1977) point out that all the pathological symptoms of this disorder may be found in normally healthy persons, so that the decisive difference is more of a quantitative than of a qualitative nature. Patients with irritable colon exhibit rapid, non-peristaltic contractions more often than do controls. Such findings occur in increased measure under stress situations and lead to disturbances in colonic function.

The personality profile of these patients is nonuniform, though it appears to include a tendency to obsessive-compulsive working over of emotional experiences when there is a depressive underlying structure (Schwidder 1965; Reindell et al. 1981). The high levels of anxiety existing in these patients has also been pointed out.

Dietary measures have primarily proved of value in treatment, and when these are combined with supportive psychotherapy the success rate appears distinctly higher.

2.4.5 Ulcerative Colitis and Crohn's Disease

Basic Aspects

The onset of ulcerative colitis may be acute and fulminant or insidious and slow. The symptoms are abdominal pain and the appearance of bloody mucous in the stools. The course of the disease may be severe and chronic or intermittent, or it may take the form of vague disturbances occurring over a period of many years. Some patients experience spontaneous remissions.

Crohn's disease is a nonspecific, chronic inflammatory disorder which usually affects the lower ileum but may involve almost all of the intestine interspaced by normal segments.

The etiology of both diseases is unclear, although bacterial, viral and immunological causes would particularly suggest that the two diseases are variants of common basic pathophysiological processes.

Personality Profile

In 60% of all new or relapsing cases of ulcerative colitis, physical signs and symptoms were preceded by life situations having depressive undertones and embodying object loss, whether real or imaginary (Freyberger 1969). According to von Weizsäcker (1951), the onset and exacerbation of the disease correlate with personal experience of disaster.

The patients come usually from families with symbiotically structured relationships in which feelings were rarely discussed. Their self-esteem is weak and they are oversensitive to failure. Particularly characteristic are their strong anaclitic desires, reflected in interpersonal relationships in which they tend to seek out persons of reference affording them such support. If such a relationship is lost, the patient unconsciously experiences the situation as a threat to his own existence. This stress situation – which may also arise from a change in occupation or loss of an accustomed environment – provides fertile ground for ulcerative colitis. The disease may also be seen as the equivalent of a grief reaction.

Freyberger (1969) cites infantility, the propensity to depressive reactions, narcissism and inhibited aggression as being characteristic of colitis patients. They lack conscious aggressive experience and behaviour yet often show strong achievement drives, even when their physical condition is greatly reduced. Elsewhere we have spoken of 'intestinal suicide' (Luban-Plozza and Meerloo 1968).

The patients restrain any form of affectivity and are consequently incapable of working through loss or separation. Such conflict is more likely to find organic expression when it cannot be verbalized. This relationship between somatization and emotional inarticulateness ('lexical lacuna') is held to exist by Marty and De M'Uzan, Fain, and Junker.

Petzold and Reindell put forward the hypothesis that patients with Crohn's disease can, along phenomenological lines, be distinguished from those with ulcerative colitis. While those with ulcerative colitis leave home relatively late and maintain the symbiotic structure of relations, patients with Crohn's disease tend to part from their parents rather early in life and the symbiotic pattern is less pronounced. Those suffering from ulcerative colitis exhibit only a slight tendency to individuation, whereas patients with Crohn's disease show a considerable capacity for introspection. A similarity has been described between the two groups of patients in that members of both usually avoid disputes and are incapable of countenancing their own feelings.

Treatment

Even in the acute stage of the disease, supportive psychotherapy is needed to supplement medication in view of the patient's frequently poor general condition and regressive attitude. This therapy is long-term and commences with attempts to build up stable object relations. Attentive listening, active counseling and specific instructions for mastering the illness form the basis of the dialogue for reinforcing the doctor-patient relationship. The aim of this ego-strengthening therapy is to promote autonomous powers and encourage competence. Owing to their marked need for autonomy, patients with Crohn's disease seem either to reject or break off treatment more readily than those with ulcerative colitis.

Petzold and Reindell (1980) stress that the long-term treatment of these patients demands a high degree of cooperation between clinical institutions and private practices. Any conflict among doctors quickly assumes a menacing aspect for the patient, who then works over the situation along the lines of object loss, which can have a very negative effect on the course of the treatment.

The combination of internal medicine and psychotherapy appears to prolong remissions, shorten the bouts of illness, alleviate pain, and help in the patient's social reintegration (Karush et al.).

2.5 Disorders of the Endocrine System

2.5.1 Hyperthyroidism

Basic Aspects

A characteristic feature of hyperthyroidism is that it often develops suddenly as a result of either strong emotion or critical situations when the predisposition exists and relevant social influences in early family life were present. Deaths, accidents and experiences of loss may not only trigger the disorder but also cause a stabilized hyperthyroidism to take a turn for the worse.

Even when apparent causes are absent, careful history taking will almost invariably uncover a particular situation giving rise to tension. Patients with a labile emotional equilibrium are likely to be associated with a complicated course and recurrences.

The frequent motoric and inner restlessness, agitation and ready irritability are sequelae of elevated hormone secretion of the thyroid. The primary purpose of these increased levels is to equip the body for extra effort over a lengthy period.

Personality Profile

We find these patients constantly prepared to overfulfill their obligations. It would appear that many of them are forced as children to become independent before they are ready; this may be because of the early death of the mother, parental separation or quarrels, early participation in family conflicts or in the upbringing of younger brothers and sisters. With significant frequency the patients are found to be the eldest of several children. They give the impression of personal maturity but this not adequate to meet all situations and only thinly veils weakness and an inner fear of separation and responsibility or of adult sexual life. Their worries may extend to survival itself, for notions of death and dying play greatly on their imagination. Alexander (1951) considered patients with hyperthyroidism to be people who had gone through a lifelong struggle to hold out against their fears.

The strong aspirations of these patients toward achievement and responsibility appear to have a self-pacifying function. According to Bräutigam and Christian, 'contraphobic' traits are found in more than two-thirds of all cases, denial and repression of anxiety in more than one-third. Four-fifths of the patients strive for advancement throughout their lifetime, their efforts to fulfill their duties leading them to the point of exhaustion. In women this is reflected as a pressing need to bring children into the world and, if possible, to adopt them as well.

Treatment

In addition to standard medical treatment, the stabilizing influence created during the consultation and working through the triggering situation at the focus of the conflict are of great value from a psychotherapeutic viewpoint. Krüskemper and Krüskemper report that the tendency of patients to react in a neurotic manner receded under standard antithyroid treatment. Consistent management by the family doctor supplemented by supportive psychotherapy can have a positive influence and reduce the number of relapses.

2.5.2 Diabetes Mellitus

Basic Aspects

Diabetes mellitus is a chronic disorder of the entire metabolism and characterized by insufficient insulin action. Although fat and protein metabolism are involved as well as that of carbohydrate, the term *mellitus* refers to the changes in blood glucose levels.

People in the industrially developed countries are at relatively high risk. Prevalence of the disease in the Federal Republic of Germany, for instance, is between 2–3%.

Over 80% of diabetics belong to the Type II group (insulin independent maturity-onset diabetes) and less than 20% to Type I (insulin dependent juvenile diabetes). The precise causes and origins of the various forms of diabetes have not been found. It is generally held for certain that a hereditary factor exists but that this alone does not lead to the outbreak of the disease. Whether this happens depends on the presence of other contributing factors, which in themselves would also not bring about the illness without the hereditary factor.

The development of Type I diabetes is probably explained by a particular disposition of the immunological system. Prior viral infections may trigger the disorder. Not only are obesity, disturbances in fat metabolism, and lack of exercise contributory factors of Type II diabetes, but also corticoids, catecholamines, and thyroid hormone (anti-insulin hormone).

Regulation of the overweight problem acquires a central significance in the prophylaxis and treatment of this type of diabetes mellitus.

Psychophysiological correlations exist in that increased release of catecholamines under emotional and physical strain inhibits the release of insulin from the β-cells of the pancreas. This in turn can lead to changes in the carbohydrate metabolism similar to those found in diabetes.

Cannon demonstrated that emotional stress can lead to elevated blood sugar levels and glycosuria by increasing sympathoadrenal stimulation. While hyperglycemia is quickly compensated in healthy subjects, this is not so in the case of diabetics.

Personality Profile

Most diabetics know that at least in one sector their homeostasis is not well regulated. They are thus troubled with feelings of insecurity. The chronic defect may exert a negative influence on their entire strategy of life. Indeed, they may organize their whole lives around this defect.

Bleuler (1975) described different personality traits distinguishing patients with maturity-onset diabetes from those with juvenile-onset diabetes. Maturity-onset diabetics do not show any particular anxiety but the presence of a certain measure of masked depression is unmistakable. Their rather open, ego-syntonic personalities tend to manifest depressive reactions when under strain. Juvenile-onset diabetics, however, may exhibit personality traits that border on schizoid features. Under strain, these patients tend to distance themselves from problems or deny them.

The psychosomatic concepts expounded in several papers on the development of diabetes were summarized schematically by Rudolf as follows:

1. Conflicts and nonoral needs are satisfied by eating. Excessive appetite and obesity may then develop and lead to constant hyperglycemia, thereby exhausting the islets of Langerhans.
2. As a result of the identification of food with love, withdrawal of affection produces an emotional experience of hunger, hence giving rise, independently of the intake of food, to a hunger metabolism which seems to correspond to that of the diabetic patient.
3. Lifelong unconscious fears result in a constant fight-flight reaction accompanied by hyperglycemia. Since no release of the psychological tension ever takes place, diabetes can develop from the chronic hyperglycemia so produced.

Despite this, there is no truly diabetic personality and these models are by no means cited as being the sole explanation for the disorder. However, particularly in juvenile diabetes, psychic factors do have considerable effect on the course of the disease and on the success of treatment. Groen and Loos ascribe special significance to the feelings of neglect and lack of security often present in these patients. Alexander describes their strongly receptive wishes for care and their attitudes conducive to dependency. Such patients develop considerable sensitivity towards the frustration of these needs, which are, analytically speaking, of an oral nature. This corresponds to the views of Reindell et al., who found that diabetics had ambivalent tendencies in their emotional life between restlessness, haste and anxiety on the one hand, and longing for peace and security on the other.

Treatment

In the course of the long-term management, patients may experience loss of autonomy and increased dependence. Feelings of helplessness and hopelessness may arise and lead in extreme cases to severe depression with a heightened risk of suicide (Reindell et al.).

According to Benedek, the risk of ketoacidosis may be increased by attempts to force the patient to diet since this can generate anxiety, conflicts and feelings of guilt. A supportive doctor-patient relationship thus forms an essential basis for prescribing a diet if treatment is to be successful.

Stabilization of the patient's emotional condition also makes it possible to achieve improved somatic equilibrium. If, on the contrary, the doctor evokes a state of anxiety and anger, this can lead to a worsening of the diabetes by reinforcing sympathoadrenal stimulation.

It might well be of advantage to consider certain psychosomatic aspects in addition to the purely medical treatment of diabetics. It is true that special psychotherapeutic techniques are rarely employed; it remains up to the physician handling the case to give the patient support; to encourage him to master life and develop new creative potential despite the cramped perspectives suggested by the illness.

However, when there is repeated metabolic imbalance a well-chosen form of psychotherapy can be of great help. The integration of these patients into a form of group therapy focusing on their illness, or admission to a hospital psychotherapeutic unit from which treatment can later be continued on an outpatient basis, has proved of great value. Family therapy is by far the best for diabetic children. Minuchin et al. showed that such families have considerable difficulties in coping with the disease, and a lack of communication between parents is often the condition immediately preceding ketoacidosis in child diabetics.

2.6 Aspects of Allergy

Basic Aspects

Allergy connotes an altered capacity of the body tissues to react to stimuli to which they have been previously exposed and become hypersensitive.

The psychosomatic approach is directed towards the psychosocial etiology of the allergic response. It is not confined to seeking out and identifying the particular allergen but in finding the nature of the previous sensitization with respect to the biographical connotation that a specific allergen has for a certain patient.

De Boor (1965) cites the example of an asthma patient whose allergen was discovered in a carpet. Although the carpet was removed, attacks recurred after the patient was discharged from hospital and only ceased altogether when the carpet's meaning for her was disclosed in the course of psychotherapy: this article of furniture had come from the house of her two sisters, whom she detested.

Another example of the connection between allergic reaction and a person's emotional condition is hay fever. This disorder has its basis not only in the hyperactivity of the nasal mucosa caused by pollen but also in the intensity and duration of the hyperemia and mucosal secretion produced by other 'aggression factors'; these include, in particular, conflict situations and anxiety states.

A fairly large quantity of allergen may therefore produce no reaction if no other stress or emotion intervenes as a precipitating factor. In other words, psychic factors can lower the sensitivity threshold to allergens.

According to Schur the disorder involves a resomatization of diffuse cathartic needs of earliest childhood, contributory factors being predisposition and environment. The psychosomatic symptom constitutes an equivalent of anxiety, and the allergen does not consist solely of a substance able to be identified by tests but also of the meaning the patient unconsciously ascribes to it.

Various skin diseases such as urticaria and eczema possess an allergic constituent. They can be vicarious disorders that replace bronchial asthma, the pathogenesis of which can also involve allergic factors. Schacht explains this phenomenon in that the skin and mucosae are nonspecific leading organs in the infant for all experience involving contact.

Personality Profile

The skin forms the outer integument of the individual. Yet although it forms an enclosure, it is open to extraneous influences. In the allergic patient the situation changes in that instead of being an 'enclosure' the skin becomes a 'disclosure'.

A characteristic feature of these patients is their complete sense of identity with their fellows. Marty gives an account of a woman patient who said she was unable to live her own life as herself but only in close association with others, as an integral part. This has its ramifications in the sexual sphere. The patient went on to say that her desire sprang from that of her partner. Marty described this form of reference structure so typical of severe cases of allergy as an allergic object relationship.

The loss of an allergic object relationship can have the following consequences:

- the seeking and finding of a new object,
- a somatic symptom,
- depersonalization.

De Boor (1965) saw that behind the protective shell of acquired adult rationality and reason, behind all the insistence on well-adjustment, loomed a larger-than-life helplessness. There was also a pressing need for lasting protection in a sheltered climate of care – an aspect of character encountered only too often in patients with serious allergies. This brings us to a personality profile that has often been described: easily hurt sensitivity hiding behind an objective, ultracorrect and often extremely rational stance against anxiety. Another facet is an affective behavioural tone with intellectually differentiated cognition.

Conspicuous traits of these patients are a sense of emotional insecurity and a continuing mother attachment. They are extremely incapable of bearing the coexistence of proximity and distance in their interpersonal relationships. The concurrence of aggressive instinctive impulses and the need to eliminate distance in their relationships appears to be characteristic. As most of these patients are inhibited in their aggressivity, they tend to keep their distance by compensatory means. This disturbance in personal and impersonal relations goes back to an earlier stage of development, to the first skin-to-skin sensations with the mother. From then onwards, the skin – whether cutis or mucosa – remained the site and theatre of action for inner conflicts.

Further aspects of allergic diseases of the skin or of the respiratory organs are dealt with in the relevant sections.

2.7 Skin Diseases[2]

The skin is particularly revealing of a person's general well-being or state of health. Indeed, it can be regarded as *the* psychosomatic organ of man, being a basis of sensory perception.

Even in the absence of any psychopathological condition, the skin is one of the most important organs of emotional expression. This is made visible when certain types of feeling and excitement produce blushing, pallor, sweating, itching, and 'gooseflesh'.

That the skin is also the site of action for inner conflicts has long been well-known and is illustrated by such time-honoured expressions as 'thick-skinned', or 'to jump out of one's skin', and 'that makes my skin crawl'.

---

[2] With the assistance of Professor A. Krebs, Director of the University Dermatology Clinic, Berne, Switzerland.

Scarcely any other organ reacts to emotional stress as quickly as the skin. It may be the integumentary appendages or the hairs that are affected.

The skin is both a barrier and an interface between the individual's internal and external world. It is an organ which can create the impression of such qualities as beauty and cleanliness, or of ugliness and repulsiveness. The skin is also a sensory organ from which stimuli are gathered and turned into such feelings as heat and cold, pain, itching and tickling, or touch and sexual responses. The reaction may take the form of circulatory changes ranging from blushing with shame to growing pale with fear, from the appearance of eczema and whealing to scale formation. It must however be assumed that there is also a predisposition to such cutaneous reactions.

Embryologists do not find these correlations between nervous and psychic factors and certain skin disorders particularly surprising. The skin and the central nervous system develop from the same germ layer, the ectoderm. Thus the skin could even be described as an 'everted' section of the nervous system – a section, however, whose functions have hardly been investigated despite the fact that this organ is more readily accessible than perhaps any other structure as an aid to diagnosis and therapy.

It is assumed that from a psychosomatic point of view the skin comes perhaps midway between organs with voluntary innervation, which are capable of giving symbolic expression to mental processes, and organs that are totally independent of volition. The latter cannot give direct symbolic expression to the meaning and purpose of mental processes.

The skin is however not only a mirror of the soul but also a medium of communication. The skin feels the longing to be stroked, and skin contact has a very direct effect on the emotional condition of a person. Those not experiencing tenderness as a child have great difficulty in extending it to others later.

This deep significance of the skin is emphasized by experience showing that massage, particularly in the nape of the neck region, can reinforce the efficacy of antidepressive drugs. The skin is thus sometimes referred to as a 'medium of therapy'.

2.7.1 Urticaria

In view of the personality aspects involved in this disorder – for which an allergic disposition must be assumed – urticaria should be seen in the same light as other allergic diseases. Musaph lists the following conspicuous personality traits of these patients:

1. a strong tendency to passive attitudes in human contact;
2. a propensity to anxiety in conjunction with a low degree of anxiety tolerance;
3. high vulnerability in love affairs;
4. a high degree of incertitude in general behaviour.

Matthes likewise stresses a behavioural aspect of these patients as being a search for object relationships of an ocnophile, clinging kind. The ocnophile has a tendency to avoid every possible risk in his search for security.

2.7.2 Pruritus

In sensitive people having a particularly appropriate disposition, strong emotions may precipitate or aggravate pruritus. It may be often observed that patients who react with irritability, anxiety and agitation under emotional tension complain far more frequently of itching and burning sensations than emotionally well-balanced people. It is moreover often found that in one and the same person evidently unaltered skin complaints itch more in periods of heavy emotional tension or of self-denial, disappointment and stress. Sexual problems, feelings of guilt, fear and anger can all evoke itching and scratching (Wittkower and Lester). It has further been observed that patients with psychogenic itching have a tendency toward a neurotic love of order and are inhibited in their aggressive impulses. Subdued anger can result in an attack of itching (Musaph).

2.7.3 Atopic Dermatitis (Disseminated Neurodermatitis)

Infancy (Infantile Eczema)

From the psychosomatic aspect this skin disorder is to be regarded as an expression of a disturbance in the mother–child relationship. Spitz maintains that his investigations have brought to light two effective factors. The infants had mothers with infantile personality structures. Towards their children they exhibited a kind of hostility that was disguised as apprehensiveness. They were mothers who did not find pleasure in touching their children or looking after them, and constantly abstained from cutaneous contact. The children for their part have an inborn predisposition for sensitive skin reactions, which means that the perceptive powers of the skin play a more intense emotional role in expression – or, analytically formulated, such reactions lead to a libidinal cathexis of the surface of the skin. Of particular importance is the ambivalent conduct of the mother. Spitz described this by stating that everything she emanates corresponds neither to her inner attitude nor to her behaviour toward the child.

This author goes on to give an example of the kind of unhealthy emotional milieu to which the infant is exposed under such circumstances: the mother avoids physical contact with her child, seemingly under the impression that she will harm it because it is so delicate and frail; such semblance of care conceals her rejection and hostility.

In many cases the disease resolves during the first half of the child's second year. Spitz thinks this may be connected with the infant's growing activity, which is then no longer solely dependent on contact with the mother but is related to things and persons of the child's own choosing.

The same author considers it is to be expected that this interlude of infantile eczema during the first years of the child's emotional development will leave lasting traces, the nature of which, however, is purely a matter of speculation.

Adolescence, Adulthood

Atopic dermatitis constitutes a pathological process within the eczematous group of diseases that is conveyed in quite a particular manner from a centre in the autonomic nervous system and is thus closely associated with patient's individual characteristics. It may occur concomitantly with other allergic disorders.

The patients frequently exhibit marked passive behaviour. They have great difficulty in asserting themselves generally. Conflicts tend to arise in their relationships with partners and are often associated with the onset of the disease. It would however appear that the patients may be split up into two groups with respect to the areas over which the inflammatory process is distributed:

- When partner relations have at least the mere appearance of remaining intact, distribution is over the flexor sides of the head and face.
- When partner relations are manifestly tense, distribution is in the region of the chest, hips, shoulders and thighs.

2.7.4 Anogenital Pruritus

Anogenital pruritus is often triggered off by local irritation, infection or some other disorder. It is characterized by severe itching, excoriation and an inflamed rash. The itching cannot always be cured by local therapy and removal of the causative irritation. Scratching and touching the itching areas becomes, so to speak, an end in itself. The pleasure derived from this activity, the resultant guilt feelings and the repeated attacks on the skin sparked off by feelings of aggression give rise to a vicious circle. The scratching can become a substitute for masturbation and often becomes a habit which maintains the presence of the symptoms and promotes their transition into a permanent condition.

2.7.5 Psoriasis

Psoriasis has a hereditary basis, but an emotional component appears to have an influence on the course of the disease. Certain nonspecific stress situations such as real or imaginary object loss, or threats to health and safety, often seem to coincide with a deterioration in the patient's condition.

There are patients who exhibit, on the one hand, such symptoms as anxiety and despondency and, on the other, those of excessive activity. It has also been observed that psoriasis patients like to display themselves in one manner or another.

Wittkower and Lester believe that the possibility of psychic factors should be considered particularly when the symptoms vary considerably and acute relapses or persistent itching occur.

However, the psychic aspect is certainly not the only relevant factor since psoriasis has been shown to be a hereditary skin disease. Even the itching is certainly not always of psychic origin but is dependent on the acuteness of the psoriasis; it occurs regularly in acute nummular episodes in adolescents. Patients with longstanding chronic forms rarely suffer from pruritis.

2.7.6 Dermatological Artifact

This refers to self-inflicted damage to the skin in the absence of any direct, conscious suicidal intent. The patients, mostly women, inflict the lesion usually when they are young. Of 35 such patients examined in the Department of Dermatology, Basel University, 27 had either at some time attempted suicide, were then undergoing psychiatric treatment, proved susceptible to occasional depression, or had a distinct psychiatric component in their family history. The psychological study clearly showed these patients to be hallmarked by considerable intrapsychic tension, severe depressive moods, inhibited aggression, strong affect-block, low frustration threshold, labile ego-integration and marked autoaggressive tendencies. Of the 35 patients, 19 had suffered from periods of depression in the past or were depressive at the time of the study.

2.7.7 Treatment

In addition to the skin disorders mentioned in the foregoing sections, many others are assumed to have psychosomatic correlations. To name but a few, there are lichen chronicus simplex, rosacea, alopecia areata and diffusa. In every case, attention should be paid to the patient's emotional state. Disturbed human relationships are frequently in the foreground. This is particularly true of skin disorders with allergic components.

The somatic reaction is in a certain sense a line of defence against the disintegration of the personality. The somatization may also be seen as an end to regression and thus constitute a possibility of building up this threatened personality. If this is attempted within the scope of psychotherapy, the strong anaclitic desire and concurrent fear of too close relationships should be worked on. Group therapy has proved of particular value in leading the patients out of their isolation.

2.8 Headache

Basic Aspects

Something like 70% of the population of industrialized countries suffer from transient headaches and about 7% from the chronic form. Approximately 10% of these symptoms arise in association with some organic cause.

Functional headaches may be diagnosed as vascular headache (migraine) or as tension headache. An attack of migraine originates from in an incipient spasmodic constriction of the cranial blood vessels. As it progresses, atony and dilatation of the arteries develop accompanied by edema, which can prolong the pain over hours and even days. In tension headache, continuous tension in the muscles of the shoulder and nape of the neck causes the pain to spread from the insertions in the cranium to all over the head.

Barolin repeatedly refers to the triad of headache, depressive moods and drug abuse.

Headaches are a common symptom in both clinical and general practice, but they occur with particular frequence in mental illness. They may be encountered in the following situations:

1. Emotional reactions to severe trauma or an acute conflict (as a psychosomatic reaction). Most of us can probably think of examples from our own experience, such as headaches after a particularly upsetting and annoying experience.

   Transient headaches can take the place of annoyance, animosity and anger. They may arise as a reaction to overtiredness and, by virtue of internal or external overstrain, as a response to a background of conflict in matters of recognition. We thus tend to find that the situation triggering off tension headache is exertion, involving some conflict in the field of achievement, when there is no possibility of inner relaxation.
2. In the context of emotional maladjustment. Here it is necessary to differentiate between simple pathological reactions where the conflicts are conscious and maladjustments in which the conflicts have been repressed.

An example of a simple pathological reaction is what Kielholz called exhaustion depression, which occurs as a result of prolonged affective strain and usually goes through three stages. In the first asthenic, hyperaesthetic stage the patients are above all irritable and extremely sensitive. In the second stage psychosomatic symptoms appear, first and foremost among which are headaches. It is not until the third stage that the true depressive symptoms finally appear as a psychic manifestation, and exhaustion of the adrenergic nervous system occurs at the somatic level (the typical depressive 'headache syndrome' in the second half of life).

Examples of emotional maladjustments where conflicts are suppressed into the unconscious are neurotic developments and psychosomatic disorders in the narrow sense. Headaches are an extremely common symptom in both forms.

3. Headaches occur in individuals with a psychopathic personality as a symptom of parathymic conditions and in stress situations.
4. Again, headaches may present as psychosomatic symptoms in endogenous psychoses.

To this category belong headaches occurring in schizophrenia. An important example is the group of symptomatic schizophrenic psychoses, including the cenaesthetic schizophrenia described by Huber, in which bizarre sensations in the head often constitute the principal symptom. Patients with this disorder frequently have difficulty in verbalizing their sensations and feelings and describe the cephalic sensations not as actual pain but rather as a strange feeling that can mount to a sense of depersonalization.

Finally, headaches are an extremely common psychosomatic symptom in depressive moods. Together with other physical complaints they can dominate the clinical picture to such an extent that the depression itself is difficult to recognize. Depression of this type is therefore often called masked depression.

Personality Profile

Neurotic mechanisms may also represent a principal factor in the etiology of the syndrome, so that the discovery of an organic lesion does not always provide the answer to the problem, as is borne out by the difficulties and inconsistent results of treatment.

Systematic investigation into the general circumstances of patients who suffer from headaches often reveals a connection between the bouts and typical episodes in the patient's life.

The psychosomatic approach sets out to find the general significance of headaches, whatever their cause may be. The headache is a troublesome obstacle to thought, and patients who suffer from it, whether migrainous or of the ordinary kind, are usually of above-average intelligence. The apparent 'neurotic obtuseness' of a large number of patients suffering from habitual headaches often seems to be nothing more than the result of thought inhibition and intellectual negativism.

Although one cannot speak of an actual 'headache type' of person, those suffering from the symptom are frequently found to have strong anxiety components, ambition, aspirations to dominate, perfectionist tendencies and the resultant chronic overstrain placed on the individual. In his confrontation with real contingencies, the high standards the patients sets himself lead to anxiety, frustration and suppressed aggressivity. This may be expressed in the basic physical deportment as chronic tension. In summary, we may speak of the patient's conflict as not being able to achieve the ends he considers desirable.

Migraine constitutes a particular form of headache characterized by a throbbing pain localized mainly to one side of the head. Other symptoms include nausea, vomiting, photophobia and concomitant neurological disturbances. The patients frequently harbour suppressed feelings which are described by Fromm-Reichmann as being a mixture of hostility and envy directed particularly against any form of intellectual achievement. He suggests that the very organ involved here could be of significance.

One could regard migraine as a form of 'swindle': it serves to conceal emotional conflicts that the patient 'need not' communicate. These patients can obtain secondary compensations from the attacks, which provide an opportunity of dominating the family and punishing their milieu in general.

Treatment

As will be clear from the above, it would be wrong simply to treat headaches purely symptomatically with analgesics when inner or external tension is present. Attention should rather be turned to the underlying conflict, which must be made accessible to treatment. This may be achieved in talks with the patient, rather in the form of short-term psychotherapy, the efficacy of which can often be increased by the concomitant use of psychotropic agents.

Both pharmacotherapy and psychotherapy can be usefully combined with physiotherapeutic measures, particularly in cases of mental disorders involving headaches. Massage of the nape of the neck is especially valuable here since psychogenic headaches, like other headaches, are usually associated with spasm of the cervicle muscles. At a later date physiotherapy can be extended to include breathing exercises and group gymnastics along the lines of 'psychosomatic training' (after Luban-Plozza).

2.9 The Sleepless Patient

Basic Aspects

Sleep protects the organism from the damaging effects of overtiredness. Under normal circumstances it follows a regular pattern, rather like hunger which occurs at habitual mealtimes.

A third of our life is spent in sleep – a considerable proportion, which would indicate its great importance to man. It facilitates vital restorative functions and relaxation. As such it should not be regarded in the light of a mere loss of consciousness but as an involuntary, autonomic regulatory process.

During sleep the body is replenished with fresh energy. One could compare the human nervous system to an accumulator of limited but flexible capacity which can only be recharged once it has run down. Sleep is thus absolutely essential to life and health in that it regularly discharges tension in one sense in order to build up potential in another.

Systematic investigations using the sleep EEG have shown that nocturnal sleep consists of stages or cycles in which the depth of sleep varies. A distinction must be made between the two major classes of sleep – orthodox and paradoxical sleep, which *cannot* replace one another. Fatigue and drowsiness are normally followed by falling to sleep, which is in turn succeeded by light sleep. Only then can the stage of moderate and deep sleep ensue, after which comes paradoxical sleep, the dream state. This undulant sequence is repeated three to five times nightly, the depth of sleep decreasing while the dream state lengthens.

The deepest sleep is not necessarily the most refreshing. Full relaxation occurs during paradoxical sleep, the phase of rapid eye movements (REM). EEG recordings have shown that during such periods brain activity corresponds more to the waking state than it does to other sleep phases, hence the term 'paradoxical sleep'. At the same time, response to external stimuli is almost zero.

Dreaming occurs during the REM phases. The eyes are in constant motion under closed eyelids, while the body is in a state of extreme muscular relaxation. The proportion of heavily relaxed phases to total sleep decreases progressively with increasing age. It is already only one fifth at the age of twenty.

Paradoxical sleep is vital to everyone. Dreams are thus part and parcel of healthy sleep, even if they are forgotten on awakening.

Probands deprived systematically of such REM sleep phases developed marked nervous symptoms even after a few 'dreamless' nights and no longer had normal reactions. During the subsequent nights of undisturbed sleep these people manifested an extreme need to 'catch up' and their time spent in dreaming was far above average. Dreams evidently relieve the mind from daily emotional conflicts. The dream would thus appear to be the indispensable handmaiden of sleep, protecting mental health just as orthodox sleep safeguards bodily health.

Sleep Disturbances

The number of people suffering subjectively from sleep disturbances increases from year to year. Between 1960 and the present day the prevalence has more than doubled. In the Federal Republic of Germany it has been estimated at 20% of the population.

Many patients complain of insomnia, generally meaning difficulty in falling asleep, interrupted sleep or nightmares. These sleep disturbances may be due to *exogenous* factors such as noise, strange surroundings, pain and indigestion. In such cases they are of acute nature and resolve when the cause is eliminated.

More difficult to counter are *psychoreactive* sleep disturbances, in which daily tensions interfere with the sleep-wake cycle. We make the following distinctions:

1. *Initial Insomnia.* Underlying this form of sleep disturbance are conflicts near the conscious level. These frequently have their roots in a neurotic development.

   The psychic tension of many patients suffering from initial insomnia is reflected in their inability to 'switch off' and to distance themselves from their anxieties, fears and everyday cares before going to sleep. Night after night, they lie awake brooding over their problems making vain attempts to abreact their 'nervous energy' that has mounted up during the course of an eventful day. The factors responsible for disturbing their sleep consist of unresolved conflicts, excessive responsibility or work load, unusual happenings or vicissitudes of various kinds. Then another threat rears its head: *the fear of not being able to sleep the next night*, which may culminate in 'bed phobia'. People suffering from this type of sleep disturbance remain tired throughout the day. But as soon as it is time to go to bed, the fear grips them – at the very sight of their bed – that they will experience another sleepless night; sleep is then prevented by their inner restlessness and agitation.

   The patient knows very well what is keeping him awake but he is unable to master the tension. Once the problems of the day have been solved, the insomnia subsides until the next difficult situation arises.
2. *Intermittent Insomnia.* The underlying factors here are conflicts well below the conscious level. When a neurotic development has reached its end point, the patient's anxious and aggressive feelings are no longer apparent to him but are expressed in his never ending brooding without awareness of the cause.

   The repressed events that have not been worked through only become apparent when the control imposed by reality has been relaxed, say, during dreams. In order to evade such emotionally stressful issues, the patient repeatedly wakes up.

   Intermittent insomnia occurring during the last third of the night is a characteristic pointer for the existence of depression. In this case the patient complains of waking up in the early hours of the morning without being able to get back to sleep again. He also mentions feeling generally in bad form mornings; this can be so marked – mostly in endogenous depression – that one speaks of matutinal or terminal insomnia.

Treatment

A sleep disturbance can be considered as a presenting symptom in the psychosomatic sense (i.e. a 'proposed symptom') once an organic cause or psychosis has been excluded. Intermittent insomnia, for example, can also occur in the presence of a tumour or degenerative alteration of the brain. Again, a latent psychotic development may give rise to initial insomnia fused with anxiety.

If the doctor simply treats sleep disturbances symptomatically by prescribing a hypnotic drug he cuts himself and his patient off from the personal aspects of the disorder. The most important question to be solved in shaping the therapy is, what daily tensions refuse to yield to sleep and why this is so.

This can be fairly quickly answered in the case of mild exogenous and psychoreactive forms of initial insomnia. It must be realized that in order to sleep well a sense of satisfaction regarding the events of the day is just as important as mental and physical tiredness. The possibility of external factors disturbing sleep should be discussed thoroughly. The afternoon nap, late meals, various sources of noise, lack of physical exercise may have become so taken for granted that the patient no longer regards them as disturbing factors.

Of great practical significance is the observation that even stimuli that fail to wake a person up precipitate reactions in neurovegetative function. This provides medical grounds for the necessity of restricting noise in the streets at night since it produces such reactions and nervous strain even when sleep is not interrupted and the sleeper is not conscious of the disturbance.

Many people who must live and sleep in the midst of busy city streets believe they have become adapted to the noise since they are only seldom awoken by sounds made outside the accustomed pattern. In reality, such people are under nervous strain and their health is accordingly endangered.

For mild sleep disturbances, in which chronic tension from conflicts is absent, autogenic training can be recommended. It owes its efficacy to the fact that those employing it for this purpose no longer attempt to induce sleep but rather yield to it involuntarily. A partial state of sleep is produced in autogenic training, which in itself is restful and restorative; moreover, the method removes disturbing elements and paves the way to natural sleep. Even more specific for this purpose is the new 'psychosomatic training'.

Severe psychoreactive initial and intermittent forms of insomnia require long-term psychotherapy aimed at revealing the conflicts present.

Hypnotic agents should only be prescribed for the shortest possible time since they do not treat the underlying disorder. One may speak of 'borrowed' sleep when they are used. As such drugs frequently suppress dream states, the patient's 'dream debt' is increased. Additional tensions and restlessness during the day followed by increased dosage or stronger drugs before retiring may induce a state in which the patient feels less and less responsible for his well-being and sleep. This can eventually lead to drug abuse.

2.10 Gynecological Disorders[3]

Many menstrual disorders, lower abdominal pain, sterility, and sexual disturbances can be understood and treated only within the general context of the patient's emotional development and affective state. Psychosomatic disorders and reactions can, however, also accompany puberty, pregnancy, childbirth, menopause, and arise as sequelae to somatic gynecological illnesses. Examinations and tests that are time-consuming, expensive, and stressful to the patient can often be avoided when psychosomatic aspects are given due consideration. Moreover, even our present day and age still bears the scars of a long tradition of hostile attitudes towards the body, under which women in particular have had to suffer. One example is described by Simone de Beauvoir: in ancient Egypt, where women were otherwise treated with great respect, confinement was enforced during the entire period of menstruation. In his work on natural history, Pliny the Elder wrote: 'The woman afflicted with her menses spoils the harvest, makes barren the garden, ruins the seed, causes fruit to fall, kills the bees; wine becomes vinegar at her touch; milk turns sour and curdles . . .' Such opinions persisted up to relatively recent times. As late as 1878 a member of the British Medical Association wrote in the *British Medical Journal* that meat went bad when handled by menstruating women. The author maintained that two cases were known to him personally where ham had gone off under these circumstances. A further example of this opinion is reflected in a regulation issued by a sugar refinery in northern France at the turn of this century prohibiting women from the premises when they had their periods. The sugar was said to turn dark. Indeed, 'the curse' is an old term for menstruation that still has certain currency.

'Somatization' covers conflicts that have not been given expression or much thought during the course of the patient's lifetime. It can have the following consequences:

1. Organic disease incurring lesions, e.g. pernicious vomiting in pregnancy.
2. Functional disorders (with physical disturbances, without organic lesions), e.g. secondary amenorrhea.
3. Physical pain (without organic damage or understandable functional disturbances), e.g. dyspareunia, backache, pelvic disorders.

The menstrual cycle begins with a folliculinemic phase, which precedes ovulation and is characterized by a gradual increase in heterosexual drives. Ovulation is followed by a lutein-controlled maternal phase when there is a more passive need to be loved and fertilized. Finally, in the premenstrual period there is a general reflux of the hormones accompanied by cleansing and expulsion tendencies.

---

[3] With the assistance of Professor M. Berger, emeritus Director of the Department of Gynecology, Berne University.

Each hormone seems to exert a specific effect on instinctual behaviour. If the drives set off in this way are not satisfied within the respective phases by sexual or maternal activity, tensions are created that throw the cycle off balance. This can give rise to a disturbance in hormonal equilibrium which in turn increases affective tension and thus creates a vicious circle with a psychosomatic content.

Disturbed partner relationships often lie at the root of gynecological disorder. Richter has provided an apt description of the course this can take in the case of a dull or taciturn husband. The dejected husband talks to his wife less and less. The wife feels hurt, loses her erotic sensitivity, and she in turn remains 'silent with her body'. Both partners withdraw from each other and both suffer by it; the husband, however, is outwardly robust and inconsiderate whereas the wife is quite obviously suffering. Her protest takes a predominantly organic form, and in the end she consults her doctor. The husband, who has remained in the background, may perhaps later accompany her to the surgery but only after repeated requests from the physician. At this point it may be possible to make the husband's sulky silence and the wife's frigidity the basis for a therapeutic discussion.

2.10.1 Dysmenorrhea

Basic Aspects

Scarcely any other field gives such scope to psychogenic and psychosomatic considerations as the female menstrual cycle. Dysmenorrhea indicates the presence of inner tensions. In some cases their connection with an actual disturbance of this type is easily recognizable, as in the case of young girls suffering from emotional strain, women engaged to be married, deserted wives, and married women who find the sexual act shameful, are unhappy at home or are afraid of becoming pregnant. In many such cases the dysmemorrhea disappears once the patient is happily married, her general conditions of life or marital relations have improved, or she finds she has conceived a hoped-for child.

Habitual dysmenorrhea, on the other hand, is often a product of deep-seated emotional conflicts. Their cause may lie in the mother's negative attitude towards menstruation, which has been transferred to the daughter. Mothers tend to speak about conception, pregnancy and birth with their daughters rather than about menstruation. The family situation at menarche is of great significance in the later integration of femininity and sexuality on the one hand, and in the development of menstrual disturbances on the other.

According to Condrau (1965) and de Senarclens (1966/68), women suffering habitually from dysmenorrhea are often those having inner conflicts. They are usually neurotic, inadaptable, frigid and consciously afraid of sexual contact. They may have masculine, active and domineering personalities, which make them feel degraded by the menstrual process. Others have remained at the infantile passive stage in their emotional behaviour: they seek maternal protection and recoil from the duties they are expected to perform as wives.

It is rare for women capable of experiencing orgasm – and have the possibility of doing so within a stable, satisfying partner relationship – to suffer from menstrual disorders. The most common cause of these disorders is infrequent sexual intercourse, perhaps once a month or even less. This is something that the patient anxiously feels she must keep a closely guarded secret. Frigidity and abstention are nearly always in evidence, as is a temporary or permanent neurovegetative tension and instinctual dissatisfaction. What was once termed 'menstrual neurosis' is nothing more than a latent form of anxiety neurosis.

The premenstrual phase is when most disturbances occur, women being anxious, irritable and depressive during this time. The nature of the disturbances depends on the fixation or regression: some patients exhibit oral dysfunctions (anorexia, bulimia, alcohol abuse), others suffer from disturbances in intestinal function such as spastic premenstrual constipation that readily changes into diarrhea during menstruation.

The importance of menstrual disorders is seen on realizing that a large number of women are condemned to suffer a form of 'menstrual invalidity' for about a quarter of their lives.

Treatment

According to Bräutigam and Christian excellent results can be obtained in treating menstrual disorders in particular by methods intended to reveal the underlying conflicts. Should the opportunity be missed of carrying out this type of therapy, an endless series of futile symptomatic and surgical treatments may follow that are not without their element of danger. Prill also recommends interpreting together with the patient what he calls 'organ language specific to the conflict'. He has compiled a questionnaire to help elucidate the subjective situation of his patients. They are asked, for example, how they feel at work, about the three persons they liked most during their youth, and about their very first friendship. This author is of the opinion that the questionnaire serves only to obtain preliminary information and that talks on more personal problems must follow. The diagnosis of a psychogenic form of dysmenorrhea or amenorrhea should not, according to Prill, be established by differential diagnosis but by examination.

2.10.2 Functional Sterility

Basic Aspects

Should a marriage remain childless despite the couple's hopes, the situation is troublesome and sad for both. Reactive depression and psychosomatic symptoms are highly frequent in such women, and the men are also affected, if to a lesser extent.

Factors playing a role in sterility include the possible tendency of some women instinctively to avoid sexual relations during the fertile period, while in other cases movements may be induced during intercourse that prevent the sperm from reaching and impregnating the ovum. It is also known that latent anxiety can cause contraction of the cervix and fallopian tubes, thus preventing the entry of the sperm. Moreover, a psychosomatic disturbance of the hormone balance can give rise to anovular cycles.

For the man's part, large variations in spermiogram parameters (sperm count, motility, morphology) correlate with stress at work and at home, so that the causes of a childless marriage must also be sought here.

Personality Profile

A truly specific type of personality has not been determined. Goldschmidt, however, has at least summarized the main personality traits as follows:

1. Emulation of masculine characteristics, overtly domineering, with a desire for independence.
2. Physically and emotionally immature with predominant dependence.

Other authors speak of a rejection of the maternal, or simply the feminine, role as being a trait of women affected by functional sterility. The psychodynamic aspects of aversion to pregnancy, birth and motherhood would appear to be associated with the early relationship to the mother.

Birbing (quoted in Goldschmidt) links the significance of pregnancy and parenthood with the relationship between the partners, between that of the wife with her own self and with the child. Provided willingness exists for conception, an intensive relationship between the partners really means that a part of the husband becomes part of the wife's self. Such 'intrusion' must be fully acceptable to a woman. The child then constitutes a kind of trinity: a separate individual, an embodiment of the child's father and of her own self.

Treatment

The primary task of the expectant mother is to integrate the growing child within her own body in order to release it later. This may prove too much for a labile personality and entail serious risk of its disintegration. The doctor should thus realize that functional sterility is possibly a means of self-protection and that its elimination can have fatal consequences.

In general practice, pointers to functional sterility emerge when psychic and psychosomatic symptoms break out in one or both partners at the same time as the woman develops amenorrhea, anovulation or follicular insufficiency. The psychodynamics involved in the unfulfilled desire to have a child can influence also the doctor-patient relationship. Richter and Stauber compared aspects of treatment in such cases:

1. Sterile couple with an 'overrated' yearning for a baby
   Degree of suffering +++ (bouts of 'child hunger', search for specialists)
   Acting out primarily by the female partner (high 'doctor turnover')
   Deterioration of the doctor-patient relationship (psychological management needed).
2. Sterile couple with a 'strong' wish for parenthood
   Degree of suffering ++ (insistence on invasive surgery)
   Depressive reactions and negative social feedback
   Can be well managed within the scope of a trusted doctor-patient relationship.
3. Sterile couple with a 'healthy' wish to have a child
   Degree of suffering + (hesitation regarding invasive techniques)
   Frustrated desire for parenthood is socially accommodated
   Harmonious doctor-patient relationship.

Goldschmidt broached the question as to whether there was any point in speaking of functionally sterile women patients instead of functionally sterile marriages. This suggests the partner relationship should be included in the plan of treatment.

The dominant pattern in the functionally sterile partnership is frequently of a clinging symbiotic nature. The relationship exhibits a stable, hierarchical order: one partner has the say, the other adapts.

Intrapsychic dynamics and interaction in partner relations must be taken into account when the possibility of extra-corporeal fertilization, which admittedly constitutes hope for many sterile couples, finds rational application.

The 'overrated' desire for parenthood, insistence on invasive surgery, the presence of concomitant reactive depression and psychosomatic symptoms, should warn the general practitioner that psychodynamic aspects need special care and attention before such techniques are resorted to.

We should like to add that psychotherapy is indicated not only in supplementing treatment of functional complaints but particularly after severe mutilating operations on the female genital tract. Such surgery can have a devastating effect on the affective and biological equilibrium of many patients and frequently causes severe identity crises. Moreover, even the prescribing of hormone therapy (oral contraceptives) must likewise be given thorough consideration because of its psychological and biological effects.

2.11 Musculoskeletal Disorders[4]

The general term 'rheumatism' includes several symptom complexes that have in common the cardinal symptom of pain in the locomotive apparatus of the body. Under this symptomatological grouping it is possible to make etiological, pathogenetic, and clinical/nosological distinctions. The three

[4] With the assistance of Dr. R. Hohmeister, Chief Physician, Medical Centre, Bad Ragaz.

main ones are inflammatory processes of the joints and spine, degenerative joint disease, and soft tissue rheumatism. A fourth group would be constituted by the 'pararheumatic' diseases, in which the pain located in tissue structures of the locomotive apparatus is indicative of another illness.

Both the social and medical implications of this group of disorders are considerable since some 5% of the population is affected. Of this, 10% are of the inflammatory type, 50% of the degenerative, and 40% soft tissue rheumatism.

The pathogenesis of musculoskeletal disorders is usually multifactorial. Immunological phenomena are involved in inflammatory processes but not in other types of rheumatism.

Experience shows that emotional factors can be of importance in both the onset and course of the disease.

Schild (1972, 1973a,b) showed that the development and exacerbation of herniated discs were influenced by the patient's *acute* emotional conflict situation. He contrasts this disease trend with that produced by the *chronic* conflict situation arising from a narcissistic personality pattern in patients with spondylitis ankylopoietica. Further psychosomatic correlations were given for inflammatory disorders, particularly for rheumatoid arthritis (see section 2.11.3).

Of particular importance in the development of arthritic disorders is the increased tone in muscle adjacent to the joints that may arise on account of tension produced by inhibited affective discharge.

The close relation of muscle tone to interpersonal communication is aptly described by Ajuriaguerra. He speaks of a *dialogue tonique* enabling two close friends or acquaintances to understand each other on certain matters without exchanging a word. The significance of emotional factors in rheumatic complaints of various origin was summed up by W. Müller as follows: 'The cause of rheumatic disorders may be psychic as well as somatic. This is particularly true of the pain in soft tissue rheumatism and, to a lesser extent, in degenerative joint processes. Inflammatory rheumatic disorders can also be modified by psychogenic factors. Therapy must take these aspects into account, and the somatic treatment should, if necessary, be accompanied by psychotherapy and/or psychopharmacotherapy.'

The displacement of the conflict to the musculoskeletal system is not restricted to any one joint. The particular localization may have a symbolic value for the patient's specific conflict.

Some idea of what is meant by 'organ language' can be gleaned from certain figurative expressions. One speaks of a 'spineless individual' and of 'persons with no backbone'.

2.11.1 Soft Tissue Rheumatism

By soft tissue rheumatism is meant a painful condition of the musculoskeletal system excluding the joints or other bone. Included are tendons, synovial sheaths, insertions of tendons, attachments of ligaments, mucous bursae, muscles, fatty and connective tissue.

Soft tissue rheumatism is not so much a diagnosis as a symptomatological collective term for pain accompanied by functional disturbance in soft tissue regions. The cause is assumed to be chronic, excessive strain of endogenous or exogenous origin on certain connective tissue. The patient's history is extremely varied, the complaints changing from time to time and influenced by many disturbing factors.

The present diagnostic criteria valid for the overall clinical picture are as follows: spontaneous pain, localized typically in the trunk and/or extremities; signs of generalized muscular pain; autonomous and functional concomitant symptoms; psychological disturbances and autonomic dysregulation.

The complaint is important in routine practice, the patients becoming a permanent problem for the doctor if he fails to recognize the psychosomatic implications. They present particularly frequently with tension in the nape of the neck. This stubborn complaint can rarely be attributed to faulty posture at work or in driving. Such a 'pain in the neck' is more likely an expression of the patient's inner tension and inability to adopt a more relaxed approach to life.

When the patients also complain of dejection and lack of drive, masked depression may lurk behind the symptoms. This diagnosis is all the more probable in the presence of concomitant sleep disturbances, palpitation, tachycardia and gastrointestinal disorders.

A conspicuous feature of these patients is their somewhat rigid way of life and high standards. Their personalities tend towards self-restraint and perfectionism. They deny themselves healthy aggressive impulses and attempt to compensate for feelings of disappointment and annoyance by 'taking a tight hold of themselves'. Their behaviour is characterized by a tendency to self-sacrifice, an exaggerated, helpful attitude that does not appear to come freely but rather from some form of inner compulsion. This attitude has been aptly described both as 'malevolent humility' and 'benevolent tyranny'.

The patient's suppressed aggressive impulses are expressed by increased muscular tension and finally by localized or generalized pain. Details given about the site of the pain may vary from one examination to another. A conspicuous feature is that the pain recedes quickly when the emotional strain diminishes.

Beck (1971) describes the patients as having strong tendencies to dependence once the disorder has broken out and that they develop a marked desire to care and be cared for. Accompanying the soft tissue rheumatism are frequently manifest neurotic symptoms, particularly anxiety states, depressive mood and psychosomatic symptoms in the form of functional cardiac disturbances, gastrointestinal disorders, headache and states of exhaustion.

The doctor–patient relationship is often endangered by the patients' ambivalent desires: on the one hand they wish to be dependent on the doctor, while on the other, despite their apparently trusting attitude, they are mistrustful and negative. The doctor has the difficult task of giving them a feeling of security and at the same time opposing tendencies towards infantilism, which considerably impair treatment.

2.11.2 Back Pain

In terms of time spent on assessment and treatment, pain and disability in the spinal region are the most important of the musculoskeletal disorders. Behind the seemingly uniform, subjective symptom of back pain lie a host of very different clinical pictures. History taking and diagnosis essentially involves all the overlapping fields of a differential diagnosis. Concomitant somatopsychic symptoms are highly frequent in patients with chronic pain. Emotional disturbances, anxiety, and repression of aggressive drives are often encountered. The following points should also be taken into account in the history taking and diagnosis: personality structure, ego strength or weakness, cultural and social milieu, even the influence of social and welfare services with all their positive and negative sides.

The patients have indisputable pain that is neither imaginary nor exaggerated. It is perhaps difficult for the doctor to accept this pain as such since there is often a discrepancy between clinical and x-ray findings on the one hand and the patient's complaint on the other. The patient may thus complain of violent pain in the absence of any objective finding. But the contrary is also possible: serious changes in the vertebrae that cause no pain are sometimes diagnosed by pure chance. Cases coming under the category of psychosomatic are those in which some psychodynamic event underlies the somatization of the disorder. The emotional conflict is no longer accessible to the patient and it is expressed by organ language.

Weintraub (1969, 1973) accorded the three main sections of the spinal column their own particular significance, which is described as follows:

Cervical Spine

In man, the cervical spine supports the head. The position of the head in humans has developed phylogenically with the attainment of an upright posture. We say that a person is 'keeping his head' or 'keeping his chin up' when he does not give way in the face of obstacles and difficulties. This effort will not lead to the cervical syndrome, so long as it forms part of a harmonious existence. Other factors, however, may give rise to the syndrome, for example emotional maladjustment, as in the case of stubborn attachment to a situation, and also chronic dysphoria where a constant extra effort of will is required to keep going. In such cases a person will obstinately attempt to achieve an aim once formulated (Blomfield 1964; Rallo Romero et al. 1969).

Thoracic Spine

The psychosomatic significance of the middle portion of the back, which roughly corresponds to the thoracic spine, is quite different. This section seems to reflect a person's mood to the greatest and most expressive degree. Grief, despair and dejection can literally weigh a man down. He says visibly and his back becomes bent. The painful muscular tension that results from this is all too often thought to be a local process of unknown origin and designated 'rheumatic' for the simple reason that the overall situation is overlooked.

A bent back in adolescents is not always due to Scheuermann's disease. In many cases it is a postural defect that has arisen because these youngsters are unable to cope mentally and intellectually with the internal and external demands made by their early physical maturity. Weintraub expressed this in words to the effect that such young people are not up to being grown up (Weintraub 1969).

Lumbar Spine

Lumbago (low-back pain) is an acute disorder. It can be triggered off by a sudden movement or by lifting a heavy object but it often occurs 'out of the blue'. In many cases spinal abnormalities such as discopathy or vertebral displacement are immaterial. Such disorders may, of course, be causative factors, but they are very often absent altogether.

Chronic lumbar pain is just as often an expression of mental strain. It is particularly common in women who compensate for their sense of inadequacy in coping with excessive family or professional demands by adopting a rigid posture, but it is also encountered in women who have ceased to resist and are weighed down by the burden of daily life with which they are no longer able to cope.

Chronic lumbar pain can also be interpreted as an expression of the frustration that arises from unfulfilled expectations in interpersonal relations and from the resultant feelings of dissatisfaction. In men this is not infrequently an unconscious admission of failure – either in their jobs or in their masculine role.

Many osteopaths, who deal almost exclusively with spinal disorders, would confirm that all 'back patients' have an emotional problem and that if there were no such problems vertebrogenic pain would virtually cease to exist.

Table 5. The psychosomatic pseudovertebrogenic syndromes (after Weintraub 1973)

Classification	Significance
1. Psychosomatic cervicalgia	Emotionally impeded self-maximation, stubborn face-saving
2. Psychosomatic dorsalgia	Grief, despair, dejection or compensatory rigid posture
3. Psychosomatic lumbalgia	Psychic overstrain, volatility, frustration, disturbed sexuality
4. Psychosomatic brachialgia	Inhibited aggression: rage, anger Symbol: clenched fist

It is important to realize that osteopaths and chiropractors owe their success not least to the close human contact – the physical contact – that links them to their patients and brings into play psychological factors of indubitable efficacy. It is also interesting that such painful conditions respond better to psychotropic drugs than to antirheumatic agents.

According to localization, Weintraub described the 'psychosomatic pseudovertebrogenic syndrome' as cervicalgia, dorsalgia and lumbalgia. He also considers psychosomatic brachialgia as belonging to this category. His classification of the syndromes and their significance are given in Table 5.

This phenomenological approach to classification is only one of several. It is also valid for 'soft tissue rheumatism'. The individual syndromes may of course overlap or replace one another according to the particular conflict or personality involved.

2.11.3 Rheumatoid Arthritis

Basic Aspects

Rheumatoid arthritis is a general inflammatory disease which can persist over years and leave permanent joint damage in its wake. Women in the thirty to fifty years age-group appear to be affected with more than average frequency.

This disease is the most important of the inflammatory rheumatic illnesses. Immunological phenomena are involved in its origin and development. A genetic predisposition is probable, but the actual outbreak of the disease is often closely bound up with emergency situations of both physical and emotional nature. Although neither the cause nor the pathogenesis have so far been properly explained, it must be assumed that rheumatoid arthritis is an autonomous disease within the general context of an immunopathological process.

Personality Profile

Not until the advanced stages of the disease do the forbearance and understanding of the patients become apparent, contrasting with the tendency of amputees to resentment and paralytics to aggressiveness. Before their illness, most rheumatoid arthritics are known for their calm and unobtrusive nature, and for being particularly capable and helpful. Striking is their altruistic attitude, which together with their energy and enterprise, makes them excellent mothers and tireless nurses. These people, who later suffer from rheumatoid arthritis, pay little attention to their own well-being and have a paucity of self-concept. Their patient, undemanding attitude contrasts with their obvious suffering; their forbearance probably corresponds to the inner inhibition of an aggression which nevertheless exists.

In the initial stages of their illness the patients are more stubborn and difficult to deal with since they cannot cope emotionally with the idea of chronicity. This is expressed by frequent changes of doctor. The intermittent nature of the disorder worries them greatly during these early stages.

In later stages they evidently come to terms with their affliction. This is admirably illustrated by Lichtwitz's description, even though it may be a little one-sided: 'Women in the later stages of rheumatoid arthritis are all very similar. There are no more kindly and forbearing patients than these. They never complain, they make no reproaches when nothing can be done for them. I always have the impression that they want to console the doctor and apologize for the fact that all his efforts are in vain. They never lose faith, they always greet the doctor with the same peaceful smile and seem to be happy when he admires the work they have done with their pathetically deformed hands. Without wishing to detract from the admiration due to such goodness, quiet kindliness and forbearance, it must be said that the moving behaviour of these patients results from a disturbance in affectivity, from the emptiness and rigidity which constitutes part of the pathological process' (Lichtwitz).

Family History and Psychodynamics

Cobb's investigations into intrafamilial influences on rheumatoid arthritis patients may be summarized as follows: The history of a woman suffering from rheumatism often reveals a weak father dominated by an authoritarian, cold, demanding mother who arouses feelings of anxiety and dependence in the patient from childhood onwards. These feelings are accompanied by forcefully suppressed rebellious urges. Being accustomed from an early age to control her own feelings, the patient tends to tyrannize those around her, from her husband, whom she chooses because he is weak and servile, down to her children, with whom she is strict and demanding. The characteristics of the male rheumatic patient correspond to those described above for women.

According to Alexander (1951) the central psychodynamic finding in such cases is a chronic inhibited, hostile rebellious state. Initially, the patients try to hold the aggression in check by exercising self-control and diverting their feelings of hatred into acceptable channels. Their need for strenuous bodily activity finds expression in increased housework and gardening and also in sporting activities. It is not until the second stage that the aggressiveness is sublimated into helpful rather than severe behaviour. The success of this behaviour is however deceptive; small incidents may easily upset the delicate balance. In particular, it becomes more and more difficult to find an outlet for the aggressive impulses. Thus, as a result of mental constraint the patient's locomotor system gradually stiffens up and is worn as a strait-jacket.

3 Psychoautonomic Syndromes

3.1 Basics

Psychoautonomic syndromes often pose considerable problems for the practitioner. Details regarding their incidence vary greatly, but roughly speaking, it is certain that at least a tenth of all young people and a third of all the patients consulting a doctor suffer from these disorders. The difficult problems arising in diagnosis and treatment are moreover reflected by the wide variety of terms employed to describe this complaint complex (Table 6).

According to Pflanz the costs for repeated diagnostic examinations of these patients are frequently some four times higher than those involved in diagnosing a carcinoma.

Patients with psychoautonomic disturbances often consult many specialists, even doctors on emergency duty, about their complaints. This frequent change of physician reflects their hope that that an organic cause will be found for their many and diverse complaints despite all previous negative findings. This places an extra burden on the medical profession and health systems alike. Moreover, the patients unconsciously try to manipulate their therapists.

Psychoautonomic disorders are defined as disturbances of the patient's state, behaviour and peripheral neurohumoural functions. Habitual or paroxysmal changes occur at the same time in all three spheres. The pathogenesis shows a uniform psychoautonomic dysregulation, the primary factor of all these syndromes.

We employ the term 'psychoautonomic dysregulation' in order to stress that not only is the autonomic nervous system involved when these disturbances occur, but that dysfunction is present. Such functional disorders have been demonstrated in tests involving this sector of the nervous system.

Table 6. Synonymous terms for autonomic disturbances

Neurasthenia	1869 Beard
Autonomic dystonia	1934 Wichman
Psychoautonomic syndrome	1934 Thiele
Autonomic syndrome	1951 Birkmeyer, Winkler
Psychoautonomic syndromes	1966 Delius, Fahrenberg
Autonomic psychosyndrome	1968 Staehelin
General psychosomatic syndrome	1981 Bräutigam, Christian
Psychoautonomic dysregulation syndrome	1982 Pöldinger

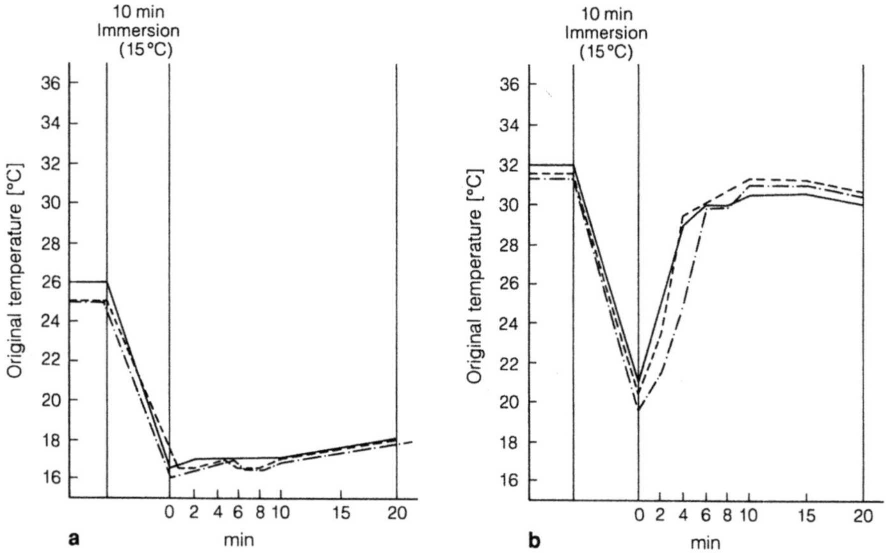

Fig. 2a,b. Cooling-rewarming test; **a** skin temperature on three fingers on a patient suffering from exhaustion depression; reduced skin temperature and impaired rewarming within 20 minutes; **b** normalization after a 2-month treatment for depression

Figure 2a,b illustrates such an autonomic functional disturbance in delayed warming up after short exposure to cold. We see how, after chilling the hand of a patient suffering from exhaustion depression in water at 15°C, a sharp fall in skin temperature ensues and rewarming to the original temperature is still incomplete 20 minutes after immersion. The same test conducted after completion of treatment for exhaustion depression showed the drop in temperature to be less and the original temperature was efficiently restored within 20 minutes. In Fig. 3a,b an orthostasis test after Schellong is reproduced showing disturbed function, which is again followed by normal results on conclusion of therapy.

Psychoautonomic disorders can occur with primary diseases of the nervous or endocrine systems, e.g. as concomitant symptoms in acute and chronic infections or allergies. They are often characteristic of the physical effects of masked depression and can arise as special forms of neurotic disorders with marked somatized anxiety. The psychoautonomic syndrome combines constitutional, exogenous-social, psychic and somatic components. The pathogenetic classification is made difficult on account of its psychogenic and/or somatogenic origin, which places it in an intermediate zone. In his attempts to establish a diagnosis, the physician may thus easily find himself in no-man's-land, which in itself can constitute a diagnostic benchmark (Fig. 4).

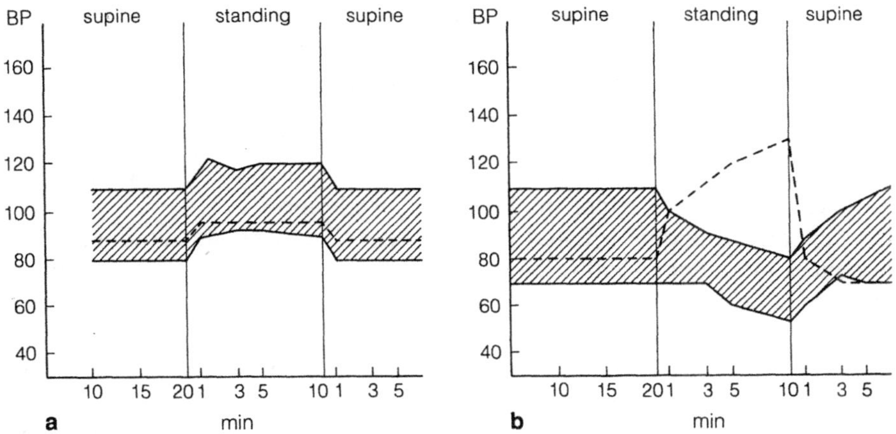

Fig. 3a,b. Schellong's test (orthostasis); **a** normal values, /// BP rise of 10–15 mmHg systolic and diastolic; .... average rise in pulse rate 16/min; **b** decompensation, /// BP drop when standing (first systolic, later diastolic) possibly until collapse; .... rise in pulse rate

	Physical symptoms	Psychic symptoms
Psychogenic origin	Organ neurosis, psychosomatic illness	Neuroses
	Psychoautonomic syndromes	
Somatogenic origin	Organic illness	"Endogenous" psychoses

Fig. 4. Classification of psychoautonomic syndromes (modified from Klussman 1986)

3.2 Pathogenetic Concepts

Autonomic reactions are normal physiological events: fear and joy alter the heart rate, we blush with shame and turn pale with fright. However, if the duration and/or intensity of the reactions becomes excessive, the state of autonomic excitability presents as a pathological phenomenon. Psychic reactions are produced that assume largely physical expression (Bleuler 1975).

Wesiack considers psychoautonomic disorders to represent alarm reactions occurring when the patients find themselves in situations they cannot overcome. With this interpretation Wesiack explains the similarity of autonomic symptoms in the prodromal stage of several somatic disorders and in unsurmounted psychosocial situations: in both cases the 'psychophysical organism lacks a suitable programme' for overcoming the emergency situation. The alarm reaction preparing the organism to fight or flee explains the occurrence of anxiety symptoms with signs of raised sympathetic or parasympathetic tone, or even a mixture of these states. If the patient is unable to reconcile the conflict, the alarm reaction can, according to Wesiack, be included under the functional syndromes.

Similarly, Kauders (quoted from Eichhorn) sees psychoautonomic disturbances as an equivalent of emotional strain that has become increasingly unbearable over the years, as persistent traumatic experiences centred around a core of insecurity and anxiety.

Delius and Fahrenberg speak of a 'potential pathogenic psychoautonomic organization' within the central nervous system. They also employ a synoptic view of somatological and psychological concepts in autonomic disturbances as their starting point. According to their hypothesis it is the weakness of the regulatory mechanism of the psychoautonomic complex in its sensitivity to situational problems that forms a basis for a type of emotional lability that predisposes to abnormal activation and inhibition alike, thus impairing the capacity to withstand stress.

Table 7 is intended to illustrate the conditions under which psychoautonomic syndromes are produced, as well as the triggering factors and manifestations.

Table 7. Conditions under which psychoautonomic syndromes are produced, as well as triggering factors and manifestations. The equivocality of these disturbances is an inevitable consequence of their origins (after Delius)

Constitutional weakness of regulatory functions (hereditary and exogenous) of the psychoautonomic complex

↓

Susceptibility to disturbances in interaction between peripheral physiological events and the CNS

↑

Traumatic experiences Conflicts Social stressors Performance stressors Noxae	Stressors	Endogenous changes Endogenous age crises

↓

Forms in which psychoautonomic syndromes are expressed

↙ ↘

Partial disturbances in autonomic function (cardiovascular, respiratory, gastrointestinal, thermoregulatory) together with emotional anomalies	Disturbances in a person's general activity (autonomic processes, sensorimotor, affectivity, cognitive processes)

From observations made on his patients, Eichhorn noted that the immediate threat posed by the autonomic disturbance was experienced as something entirely 'anonymous'. It was like a confrontation with an unfamiliar function apparently existing outside the normal personality but paradoxically experienced as one of their own body functions. On several occasions patients had expressed the feeling that a process was developing strictly in accordance with its own laws, against which they were helpless. In somatic aspects, Eichhorn interprets his observations along the same lines as Wesiack when he compares the reactions of patients with those of other people in sudden, life-threatening situations, namely, their inhibited conscious processes, which open up the way to instinctual behaviour and autonomic reflex activity.

Eichhorn views psychoautonomic disturbances under the aspects of Dasein analysis. He relates the apparent independent course taken by the autonomic event to the patient's scheme of life, which is marked by excessive strivings for autonomy at the expense of inherent and natural powers of transcendence. According to this author, such a disturbance in the patient's scheme finds continuation not only in autonomic events but also to a certain extent in basic life processes. In other words, the loss of meaning can lead to a loss in meaningful organic function.

3.3 Triggering Factors and Personality Profile

In adults, psychoautonomic syndromes usually occur between the ages of thirty and fifty, a period when pressures of work are at their greatest. The patient's case history often reveals ambitious strivings, a hectic work situation or general dissatisfaction with the type of work.

Seemann listed behavioural factors common to patients presenting with functional disturbances in the cardiovascular system. He comments on finding a form of behavioural lability both in physical events and interpersonal relationships. The patients set themselves or accept targets, but their general lack of self-assuredness prevents the necessary action getting under way. They fall between two stools (Seeman quoted from Staehelin 1963).

General factors belonging to the sphere of individual psychology and biology that are responsible for triggering phenomena of autonomic excitation include:

Disturbances in the sleep-wake cycle;
increased pace of life;
overexposure to stimuli;
increasing loss of ideals and growing materialism.

The following special factors belonging to the sphere of object relationships can result in autonomic disturbances:

Financial worries;
isolation, uprooting, lack of human contact;
love or sexual conflicts, lack of recognition;
excessive strain in working mothers;
particular problems in bringing up children;
conflicts at work;
overwork.

Such preconditions are often encountered in persons of a quiet, unobtrusive and reserved nature, who develop unmistakable depressive-compulsive traits and a hypochondriacal attitude towards their symptoms. The patients persistently describe these symptoms, sometimes in dramatic detail.

The psychodynamic picture is frequently one of a marked dependency/autonomy problem complex originating from an unsatisfactory and disappointing relationship to childhood persons of reference. Tendencies towards independence and expansive impulse are usually suppressed and replaced by a fear of separation which cannot be resolved but only somatized as the disorder develops.

As Staehelin (1969) observed in a study on 600 patients, the loss of inner security, of the fundamental confidence normal to man, generally heralds the onset of an autonomic syndrome. In view of the great number of people suffering from autonomic dysregulation, he declared that this lack of basic confidence was the commonest psychopathological symptom of our time.

3.4 Types of Decompensation

If, owing to their life styles, people are exposed to an excess of afferent stimuli, the reticular activating system may be unable to cope and autonomic decompensation will occur. This takes place in two stages:

1. An autonomic-affective excitation syndrome. Cardinal symptoms are irritability, tenseness and anxiety.
2. An autonomic-affective exhaustion syndrome characterized by fatigue, exhaustion and depressive mood.

According to Willi (1975), the persistence of general tiredness even after a lengthy period of sleep is due mostly to an underlying paradoxical situation. The author goes on to explain this in words to the effect that the patient produces work that he does not admit goes against the grain.

A whole range of ancillary complaints may also be present: sleep disturbances, tingling inside, restlessness, constant agitation, sweating, loss of appetite, palpitation, headache, dizziness and a general feeling of uneasiness.

3.5 Treatment

The patient is irritated by the intensity and multiplicity of his complaints, and the somatically oriented physician loses confidence when the search for pathological findings proves unsuccessful. Moreover, the usual prescriptions of drugs cannot by themselves keep the autonomic reactivity under lasting control. A fruitless search for physical disorders serves only to intensify the patient's feeling of illness and the resultant anxieties.

The majority of these long-term, endogenous syndromes have a good prognosis. They do, however, place a strain on the patient's behaviour, health and way of life. They do not endanger life, but usually prove resistant to attempts at a lasting 'cure'. These patients are 'incurably healthy'. Over half of all psychoautonomic disorders are of this chronic recurrent or primary chronic type.

Psychoautonomic disorders are never dangerous, however unpleasant they must seem to the patient and however great the burden on the general practitioner. The doctor must convince the patient of this without, however, giving the impression that his complaints are of no real consequence; for a prime condition of the treatment is that the patient must feel he is understood and accepted.

The situation is somewhat different where highly localized syndromes are concerned. Psychoautonomic disorders that affect the gastrointestinal tract can pave the way for ulcers or ulcerative colitis. A hypertensive regulation disturbance can sometimes develop into essential hypertension.

One of the doctor's most important therapeutic functions consists of listening to the patient. Empathy will prove of more help to the patient than many attempts at giving advice. Listening is in fact absolutely essential for understanding patients and their problems. Only then is the doctor in a position to decide whether they can best be helped by either psychotherapy, a series of advisory and supportive talks, or a change in milieu.

We agree with Wesiack that even discussing these possibilities makes a considerable, initial contribution to therapy. It may be that the patient then already begins to recognize certain connections of which he was hitherto unaware. This may kindle desires to change things or adopt a possible course of action.

According to Beck, a suitably trained family doctor may take in hand the psychotherapy himself when the following criteria are present:

1. The patient must be conscious of the conflict and have at least an inkling of how the functional symptoms are bound up with his own life and that they do not constitute events alien to his ego. The most favourable situation is the presence of an acute, real conflict concurrent with the functional symptoms.
2. Functional symptoms associated with anxiety – better suited to psychotherapy than are hypochondriacal complaints.

3. The functional symptom should not date back more than one year. With increasing duration, processes set in that render psychotherapy difficult (e.g. iatrogenic fixations or habituation to secondary gains derived from the illness).
4. The patient should feel a need to talk things over with the doctor and be able to draw conclusions from such discussions. A prime condition is the patient's active, inner cooperation. It is not enough for the patients to submit themselves passively to questioning and persuasion – and expect that the mere compilation of facts about their lives will effect a change for the better.

4 Psychosexual Disorders

4.1 Basics

The frequent tendency of patients today to consult their doctor about sexual disorders is undoubtedly related to the increasing openness shown toward sexual matters in general. Yet freedom in this domain has brought about not only advantages. Greater knowledge and wider opportunity very easily lead to attitudes in which personal commitments of this kind are regarded in the light of sexual 'performance', and it is particularly under such pressures that failure is encountered. These pressures and concomitant fears of not coming up to expectations are the most frequent causes of functional disturbances; such factors are generally found to constitute an ominously linked reaction in which fear of the symptom leads to the symptom.

The other side of the coin is that research and progress in this field have opened up new and more efficacious methods of treatment in a relatively short span. Figuring among the new methods that have recently proved of particular value in treating this group of disturbances are behavioural therapy, client-centred therapy along the lines of conjoint therapy and focal short-term therapy. Special mention should be made of the pioneer work of Masters and Johnson which has paved the way to new strategies in treatment. One important advance is in treating the couple always jointly. In the original method advocated by these authors, the couple were treated by two therapists, one male and the other female. Their method has been employed in Europe mostly in a simplified form with only one therapist.

It will already be realized from this introduction how important it is for children to be informed correctly on the 'facts of life' and receive sex education. However, young people apperceive not only from what is presented to them in the form of verbal communication but also from averbal forms or, as in this case, difficulties in communication on the part of the parents.

The most frequent sexual disturbances encountered in medical practice among men patients are impotence and premature ejaculation, while the order of importance of those found in women patients would be libidinal disturbances, then dyspareunia and lastly anorgasmia.

4.2 Pathogenic and Therapeutic Concepts

The various theoretical approaches forming the basis of methods of treatment for functional sexual disturbances are as follows:

Informatory	→	Explanatory information, counseling
Learning processes	→	Behaviour therapy
Communicative	→	Client-centred therapy
Psychodynamic	→	Psychoanalysis
Existential	→	Dasein analysis Logotherapy

As previously mentioned, various sexual disturbances can be traced to a lack of necessary explanatory information. Also important are the approaches based on learning theory, which have led to the invaluable employment of behaviour therapy in this field. Such approaches are based on the theory that a certain sexual experience was, for example, coupled at one time with very disturbing events, the sequel being that whenever sexual excitation is awoken anxiety occurs. This inhibits normal intercourse. Impotence is thus in many cases caused simply by the fear of repeated impotence.

The significance of the communicative approach becomes apparent on reflecting that the sexual act represents one of the most important forms of averbal communication in interpersonal relations. These are very easily disturbed when verbal and general communication is impaired. It is, however, often very difficult to decide in individual cases whether the sexual disturbance is a sequel to impaired communication or whether this is a consequence of the sexual disturbance. This is where client-centred therapy plays a useful role and may even achieve a cure.

Psychodynamic approaches and depth psychology continue to have great importance since it is often a case of repressed conflicts leading to complexes that exert a strong, unconscious influence and result in severe sexual disturbance. The patient is naturally unaware of such ramifications, which can only be brought to light by psychotherapeutic, particularly psychoanalytical, techniques and thus rendered ineffective with respect to the disturbance. It should be mentioned in this context that short-term therapy has proved to be of particular value in sexual disturbances. Even Sigmund Freud, whose attitude towards short-term approaches was critical to say the least, succeeded in ridding Gustav Mahler of his impotence after a mere three sessions.

Finally, mention must be made of the no less important philosophically orientated approach of Dasein analysis. This group also includes logotherapy developed by Viktor E. Frankl, to whom we owe the concept of paradoxical intention, which was later taken over by behaviour therapy.

4.3 Forms of Treatment

The list at the beginning of section 4.2 summarizes possible ways of treating psychosexual disorders.

Directive Counseling

Should we commence with this educational approach, it is important to realize from the outset that many sexual disturbances arise from the ignorance of both partners regarding the different sexual response cycles in man and woman. This curve was first plotted by the gynecologist Kafka. Fig. 5 reproduces the somewhat more recent version after Duss-von Werth and Hauser.

We see that the excitatory phase progresses rapidly in the male and that after a short plateau phase the climax of the sex act is achieved in ejaculation. Sexual excitation then very quickly resolves. In contrast, the excitatory phase of the female rises very slowly up to a lengthy plateau phase, and after orgasm excitation diminishes likewise slowly. It is thus of great importance to make men aware of the inadvisability of immediate penetration of the vagina. They should be advised to stimulate their partner slowly into the right mood of sexual excitation and restrain themselves for some time before direct intercourse.

Once this has commenced, care must be taken that the woman also achieves orgasm. Should ejaculation occur before this and penile erection subside, or the man is unable to continue coitus for other reasons, it is important that the female partner is brought to her climax by other means, e.g. manual stimulation. Even afterwards the man should continue to express his tenderness until her excitment has abated.

Figure 6 shows possible courses taken by both sexual response cycles. When they are not in harmony mutual satisfaction will be absent. It is also very important to mention within this context that various types of foreplay by all means have their place in forming the individual hallmark of person's sexuality; the idea is quite wrong that everything not pertaining directly to coitus in the usual position is a perversion. This includes the important question of varying the positions, which is certainly not just a topic for pornographic literature. Such variations can heighten erotic feeling and

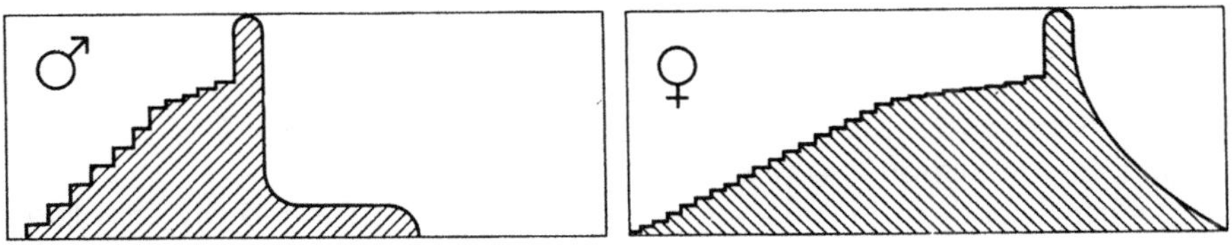

Fig. 5. Male and female sexual response cycles (after Duss-von Werth and Hauser)

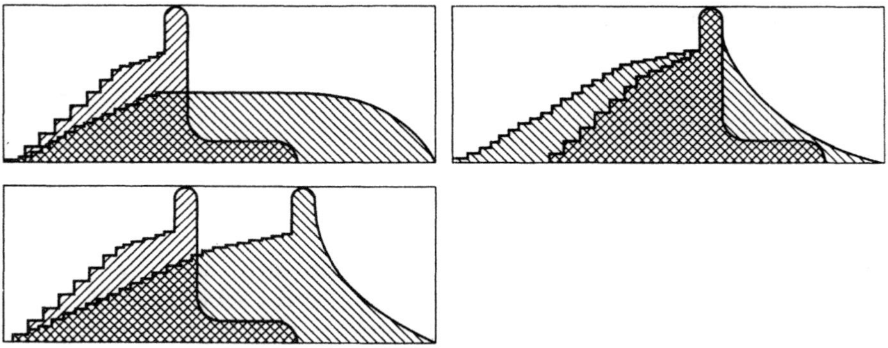

Fig. 6. Superimposed male and female sexual response cycles illustrating disharmony and harmony (after Duss-von Werth and Hauser)

strengthen the ties of affection in an intimate relationship of this kind. It should be emphasized that one can speak of a perversion only when it constitutes the sole means of gaining sexual satisfaction. As long as the act is merely an elaboration of normal intercourse and ultimately leads to normal satisfaction with the normal sexual object one usually speaks of variations in lovemaking, provided they remain part of a pleasurable, mutual experience and do not give rise to aversions.

Abstention from Intercourse

A second method of treatment consists of instructing the couple to abstain from intercourse for a certain time. This initial restriction is important in that the focal point is then no longer the disturbance itself but the doctor who has imposed the ban. Attempts are usually made to deviate from the restriction and in the ensuing discussion between the partners, and exchanges of endearments or caresses, it often happens that intercourse suddenly becomes possible again. This is because the sexual disturbance itself is forgotten in breaking the imposed abstention.

Autogenic Training

As sexual disturbances are usually accompanied by tenseness, autogenic training constitutes a very apt method of treatment. The patient can, for example, distance himself from his incapacity by repeating to himself a phrase such as 'I just couldn't care less about my disorder'. This also produces dereflexion and thus leads to relaxation.

Such exercises in relaxation can also be performed by Jacobson's methods. In this technique a series of different muscles are strongly tensed then suddenly released. Under this state of sudden muscular relaxation it is impossible to experience anxiety, albeit for a short time. Relaxation exercises consequently form an important part of behaviour therapy.

Client-Centred Therapy

This form of treatment is important since sexual disturbances are frequently a problem of disturbed interpersonal relationships. In the narrow sense we may speak of a therapy centred around aspects of communication, or conjoint therapy when – what is absolutely necessary – both partners take part in the talks and not only the one who first sought treatment. In therapy employing depth psychology the aim is to make conscious repressed conflicts that have become unconscious complexes, and as such have disturbed sexual relations by, for example, bringing into play inhibitions and symptoms of anxiety. It is important to realize, however, that this aim can be achieved not only within the scope of long-term psychoanalysis but often by focal therapies. These employ the general approach of depth psychology but concentrate on a specific problem.

The most important analytic problems encountered in male and female psychosexual disturbances are given in the following listings, which have been modified from Becker.

Analytic Aspects in Male Psychosexual Disorders

Impotence	*Castration complex*: fear of retaliation *Oedipus complex*: continual competition with supposed rivals *Fear of aggressive components* in own sexuality
Premature ejaculation	*Oedipal attitude idealizing* the wife: not to injure, not to give *Urethral fixation*: disinclined to 'give' (in the sense of fertilization)
Unduly delayed ejaculation	*Feelings of guilt* prevent pleasure Reluctant to give (e.g. his semen) due to castration complex, with fear of ego loss, in orgiastic regression (death anxiety)

Analytic Aspects in Female Psychosexual Disorders

Oedipus complex	Doting affection for father complicates later partner relationships; aggressive father causes regression to oral phase
Problems of female identity	Penis envy leads to projection of phallic omnipotence on the partner, who does not come up to her ideal
Ego weakness	Fear of ego loss in orgiastic regression (loss of control) leads to shame and anxiety
Female sadomasochism	Destroys every possibility of normal sexual function

Dasein Analysis and Logotherapy

A large proportion of sexual disturbances can be treated from the Dasein analytical and logotherapeutic aspect, particularly in patients for whom the sexual disturbance is the expression of a general life crisis. Of especial importance in logotherapy is the method of *paradoxical intention*, followed by dereflexion since many disorders persist because they are the object of too much reflection. It can be said for the simpler forms of both client-centred therapy and methods involving depth psychology that they are not in the strict sense merely the domain of the psychoanalyst. It is quite possible to acquire the necessary therapeutic armamentarium for carrying out simple psychotherapy by, say, participating in Balint groups and having a check made on the first few treatments.

It should perhaps be stated at this juncture that although there should be specialists and research centres for sexual problems, this does not mean that a new specialty or discipline should be created. On the contrary, knowledge of the sexual aspects of medicine together with psychotherapeutic know-how and experience should be made as widely available as possible for every doctor to use in his practice. The trusted family doctor in particular is the most likely person to whom people with sexual difficulties will turn for help. It must moreover be realized that almost everyone finds it difficult to talk about sexual problems. It is thus very important that such specialists as gynecologists, for example, include questions regarding the patient's sexual behaviour in routine case history taking.

Behaviour Therapy

The widespread and erroneous assumption that the doctor's chances of learning psychotherapeutic techniques are limited is particularly untrue of behaviour therapy. Enough know-how to conduct simple investigations and apply such therapy can be acquired by attending relatively short courses.

Without attempting to cover all the problems involved in behaviour therapy, we should nevertheless like to present a few examples of its application in sexual disturbances. Behaviour therapy consists of attempting to dislodge certain ideas and conceptions from the anxiety with which they are bound up, along the lines of desensitization for example. Treatment of the anxiety is by relaxation exercises, whether by those prescribed by autogenic training or those of Jacobson's progressive relaxation described below.

The latter consist in strongly contracting certain muscles followed by conscious awareness of their relaxation. The author has compiled an extensive list of individual muscles that can be contracted and decontracted. The following is a simplified version:

Press eyelids together;
press lips together;
press the chin against the chest;
clench fists;
tense the biceps;
press the elbows against the ribs;
contract abdominal muscles;
contract the muscles of the pelvic floor;
press the knees together;
in a sitting position, brace the toes against the ground.

These relaxing exercises also play an important part in what is known as desensitization, one of the methods of modern behaviour therapy that has found wide application in psychosexual disorders.

In the moment of full physical relaxation it is impossible to experience anxiety, and advantage is taken of this phase to separate sexual experiences associated with anxiety from the anxiety component. In order to do this, however, we must first compile a 'hierarchy' of the ideas producing the anxiety. The patients themselves are asked to make a list of all such ideas. These are then sorted out into an order of priority, beginning with the ideas eliciting the most anxiety.

An attempt has been made in the listing below to summarize such a hierarchical conception. At the very bottom of the list are the erotic allusions and entering the bathroom, which already evoke anxiety, and topmost are the actual penetration of the penis and intercourse. This was the hierarchical anxiety pattern of a woman patient suffering from dyspareunia.

Intercourse
Penetration
Opening the legs
Clitoral stimulation
Touching
Observation
Fondling of the breasts
Undressing
Embracing and kissing
Entering the bedroom
Bathroom
Erotic allusions

After this was compiled, the patient learned the relaxation exercises and, starting from the bottom of the list, was asked to imagine these situations. As soon as it became possible for her to think of one of these situations without experiencing anxiety, she was allowed to proceed to the next. The exercises are initially supervised, after which the patient may perform them alone.

Following the desensitization 'in vitro', so to speak, it is then quite possible that the couple will continue it 'in vivo'. It is essential that the partner is well informed and prepared to cooperate, particularly in the sense that he is willing to interrupt intercourse when the other partner becomes anxious and not resume until later when renewed relaxation has dispelled anxiety.

However, fears connected with sex do not arise singly in most cases but are accompanied by others, particularly in neurotic patients. It is thus important to compile in addition a hierarchical pattern of nonsexual fears in the same manner. This has been done below:

Death of a near relative
Disturbing news
Having to speak with strangers
Walking alone through dark streets
Driving a motor vehicle
Not coping with household duties
The husband must suddenly leave on a journey
Cardiac infarction
Crowds
Cable cars
Air travel
Cooking stove not turned off.

Combined Therapy

According to our experience it is advisable to treat sexual disturbances initially by the methods described earlier in this chapter – i.e. by explanatory information, paradoxical intention and abstention from intercourse – then by behaviour therapy. Once the symptoms have disappeared, however, attempts should be made to get to the root of them by an analytical approach. Such combined therapy has proved valuable since behaviour therapy is eminently suitable for eliminating the symptom, while light can be shed during the course of interview therapy on unconscious processes, particularly if the approach has a bias towards depth psychology.

Much has been published on the methods of Masters and Johnson, notably in the lay press. The essentials of their treatment are summarized as follows:

Separate talks and examination
Joint round-table discussions
Explanation
Discussion on conflicts
Practical modification of behaviour by sensate-focus-oriented therapy
Round-table check-up talks on progress.

Although the method of Masters and Johnson has a bias towards behaviour therapy, it also contains elements of client-centred therapy. The essence of their treatment is the employment of two therapists working as a team. Discussions are initially held individually with the two partners, then with the couple and both therapists. The important phases of these talks are first of all explanatory and informative, then revelatory with respect to conflicts, followed by behavioural approaches. As previously stated, the partners are instructed how to overcome the disturbance 'in vivo' by employing aspects of behaviour therapy, particularly that of desensitization. This method has been notably successful in the United States.

We conclude with a few words about the success of the various methods of treatment discussed here. Just as it is difficult to grasp the true nature of sexual disturbances, it is not always easy to obtain a critical evaluation of the success achieved, particularly in modifying the behaviour of anorgastic and frigid women patients. A listing has thus been drawn up in the form of basic questions which can be posed, especially to women, in order to elicit the degree of success achieved by the therapy.

Do you look forward to having intercourse?
Do you nearly always have an orgasm?
Do you ever take the initiative in sexual activity?

The methods discussed here of treating sexual disturbances surely indicate that no great difficulties stand in the way of acquiring in relatively short time the necessary armamentarium for use in present-day medical practice. We are of the opinion that the treatment of sexual disorders is a very worthwhile concern of medical practice; in this age of meritocracy it is important to resist the tendency to regard our patients and successes solely in the light of making people fit for work when it is equally important to render them capable of love in their private lives.

4.4 Sexuality with Increasing Age

Women of increasing age constitute a particular problem and concern in this field of medicine. The menopause is still experienced as something rather dreadful, and often felt to be a loss in status and esteem. This can be attributed to inadequate explanation and reassurance. Many women nurse the belief that the onset of menopause spells the end of their capacity for sexual love and enjoyment. Women who have undergone hysterectomy are troubled by similar fears. In reality, the uterus is essential neither for libido nor for orgasm. Masters and Johnson have defined orgasm in the woman along the following lines:

1. Sensation of suspension or stoppage. Lasting only an instant, the sensation is accompanied or followed immediately by an isolated thrust of intense sensual awareness, clitorally oriented, but radiating upward into the pelvis. Intensity ranging in degree from mild to shock level has been reported by many women. A simultaneous loss of overall sensory acuity has been described as paralleling in degree the intensity and duration of the particular orgasmic episode.
2. A sensation of 'suffusion of warmth', specifically pervading the pelvic area first and then spreading progressively throughout the body.
3. A feeling of involuntary contraction with a specific focus in the vagina or lower pelvis. Frequently, the sensation was described as that of 'pelvic throbbing'. The initial contractile feeling was described as localized vaginally, subsequently merging with the throbbing sensation which, though initially concentrated in the pelvis, was felt throughout the body.

From the aspects of both sexual and mental health it is important that women are given a timely explanation that neither menopause nor hysterectomy means the loss of their lovelife or of their capacity to have an orgasm. The libido may even increase initially during menopause. This often has an anxious effect on women who expect a decrease in libido. Its increase occurs as a result of a reduced secretion of female sex hormones giving rise to a relative predominance of male sex hormones, which are also produced in the female adrenal cortex. Frequent sequels are the first signs of facial hair and a deeper voice, which constitutes a special problem for singers.

The answer as to how long a woman can enjoy sexual intercourse is simply: as long as she has or can find a partner. The capacity for sexual love in the woman is thus less dependent on age than in the man insofar as the ability and not the opportunity is concerned.

It is particularly important that gynecologists bring these circumstances to the attention of women who are about to undergo major surgery such as hysterectomy. It is interesting to note that this psychological element is sometimes forgotten. Substitution therapy invariably comes to mind in connection with oophorectomy; this is also doubtless a consequence of the somatic orientation of the conventional medical curriculum, which is now happily acquiring an extension in a new, psychological dimension (Pöldinger 1987)

4.5 Personal Experience of the Consultation in Psychosexual Medicine

Research into sexual disturbances and the methods of treatment developed from it have made great progress in recent years. The onset of this trend coincided with the removal of certain taboos and a general liberalization in sexual matters. Patients began to consult their doctors about their complaints and request treatments that were then available for some 80% of psychosexual disorders. There nevertheless still appear to be liminal fears on the part of doctors and patients alike. It costs much effort for many patients to discuss their sexual problems.

The doctors' inhibitions in this respect spring from a frequent belief of not being equal to the situation, neither emotionally not from the standpoint of training. We can at least say, however, that today there is no shortage of literature in this field for putting oneself in the picture. Then of course there are the Balint groups. These provide the opportunity of breaking down the emotional difficulties and bringing awareness that the relationship between patient and therapist is here the key factor instead of merely the clinical findings. A successful group orientated along these lines has now been in operation for eight years at the Women's Clinic of the University Hospital in Basle (within the framework of the Social Medical Unit and Family Planning). This particular Balint group consists of a core of regular members, colleagues in other departments and various members of the medical profession who seek training in this field for a limited time. Experience has shown that the participants are able to take over certain cases needing explanatory information and treatment within a relatively short time.

In reviewing the various patterns followed by consultations in the field of psychosexual medicine that have primarily developed during the last ten years, it is possible to draw the following conclusion: although based on different therapeutic concepts, there has been a comparably similar development in individual consultations with respect to methodology. In other words, the different concepts were able to be brought into line, whether they involved client-centred therapy, behaviour therapy, short-term psychoanalytical therapy or the general-systems theory. The overlap of methods used by Masters and Johnson must also be viewed in this light. It is also interesting to note that various syntheses were attempted in treating psychosexual disturbances in order to unite behavioural and psychodynamic approaches. This appears understandable on reflecting that, for example, ignorance of causal relationships can on the one hand be regarded as repression and on the other as the sequel to a defective learning process in the sense of faulty conditioning. Indeed, psychosexual disorders arising in this manner may also be conceived as a form of communication disorder, and therapy along these lines may be very successful. Research in communication has enriched the choice of methods available. Another reason for improved results in therapy is that in the main the partners are only treated jointly; in the original method developed by Masters and Johnson two therapists were employed, whereas in Europe this is only practised in very difficult cases.

5 Psychological and Psychosomatic Aspects of Dentistry

M. Fisch[5], Lugano

5.1 Basics

After its historically conditioned emphasis on manual and mechanical skills, dentistry became increasingly orientated towards basic research findings in the biological sector. This development caused the profession to model itself more and more along medical lines and acquire sharper definition from dental technology. Moreover, despite their work being confined to the stomatognathic system, dentists were obliged by this trend to obtain better insight into the importance of both organic and psychosomatic correlations.

Preventive dentistry is an excellent example of the increasing importance of psychology in practising a profession, not merely from a technical viewpoint, but out of social and ethical considerations too.

Not so very long ago, the dentist was considered a manually skilled specialist, who either alone or together with a dental mechanic, restricted his work to restoring functional and cosmetic aspects. Today, he must devote more and more of his energies to the prophylaxis of caries and periodontal problems (Swiss Dental Association 1986).

Check-ups, inventories, scaling, and continually motivating the patient in questions of dental hygiene and self-discipline with regard to food, must also be mentioned as belonging to the present spectrum of activities. There are a host of others the dentist can no longer carry out on his own, and in many countries this has led to adding a hygienist and a dental assistant to the staff. Help is also needed in administration. The management and coordination of this team demands a degree of skill and tact not exactly innate in everyone.

Although even the old-time dentists considered patient-specific explanations the best means of ridding their 'victims' of the dread of the treatment to come, it is now also the duty of the dentist, legal obligation in many countries, to inform the patient of any possible risks involved. This, as well as the prophylactic motivation mentioned above, is not always easy, particularly from the psychological point of view.

The radical changes taking place in our work and way of life have, in the wake of unprecedented technological progress, made grave inroads on

---

[5] With the assistance of E. Strich-Schlossmacher.

man's physical, emotional and mental equilibrium. This is manifested by the increasing number of emotional disorders and interpersonal conflict situations.

On the one hand, they influence the relationship of the dentist to the state and bureaucratic authorities, who, via the various health insurances, tend to wield more and more sway over his erstwhile freedom. On the other, they have affected his contact with the ever more important assistants in the practice; even more affected are the patients: their attitudes toward their oral situation, their trust and expectations regarding treatment, as well as their readiness to share inevitably in the responsibility for dental health.

These changes are becoming the growing cause of disturbances in mind-body interactions and diverse, related organic dysfunctions, which may also arise in the maxillofacial region. Typical of this situation are increases in mandibular joint disorders in recent years – not, let it be remarked, due entirely to improved diagnosis – and prosthesis intolerance, which is only too well-known to every practitioner.

It is thus becoming of additional importance for the dentist to recognize the reasons for his patient's behaviour and be aware not only of the technical responsibility involved but of human obligations too.

To the dentist receptive to new ideas it will appear that his profession has reached a point where it will have to attend more to emotional factors than technical innovations (Kleinknecht 1976). Such impressions have in fact already given rise to special training producing 'psychodontists' or dental psychologists. These graduates are naturally more versed in behavioural and psychological aspects than their colleagues and better equipped to deal with the age-old problem of fear and the indifference shown towards hygienic and prophylactic measures (Leatherman 1978). When we take all this into account it does indeed seem a far cry from the days of the barber-surgeon. Our image, like that of the medical profession, has everything to gain by this trend in the direction of holism (Holz 1978).

Awareness of the relation between defective teeth and emotional reactions is nothing new, but it tended to find representation more in humorous folklore than in scientific literature. Wilhelm Busch, the German artist and writer of comic verse, expressed this aptly in *Balduin Bählamm*. His style is inimitable but a free translation would be along the following lines: 'Only in that narrow hole/Of the backtooth bides his soul/Till in writhing does he shout/The tooth must out!' Yet Busch does not let the matter rest by describing merely the patient's emotional state but gives the dentist a certain measure of psychological understanding by having him say: 'Now lean your head upon this rest/And only think of all that's best!' In this satirical verse 'The Hollow Tooth' several aspects of the problems involved in dentistry become apparent: at the other end of a single tooth is a whole person with all his physical and emotional troubles; there is the fear of the dentist, which keeps the patient away from having an urgent examination until pain gives the alarm; and even when he finally makes his way to the surgery it is perhaps not until he has tried every possible household remedy. The continuing and repeated attempts to take the edge off the more unpleasant aspects of dental treatment by humorous approaches have been recently illustrated in a noteworthy thesis by Bernheim.

5.2 The Significance of the Oral Region

The mouth and lips belong to the highly intimate parts of the body; they are thus directly bound up with feelings and hence invested with a high degree of affectivity, both in positive and negative aspects. Intervention in this region is experienced as something very personal, and the dentist's personality is accordingly of great influence (Reisner 1972).

Psychological studies have shown that the importance attached to the teeth is to some extent rooted in an elemental symbolism of strength, of potency in the broadest sense, and in aesthetic values, which extends far beyond that of their anatomical structure and function. This symbolic significance is comparable to that possessed by the hair, and as one of the crowning signs of health and perfection influences intrinsic aesthetic values and hence related feelings of physical and emotional well-being (Dolder 1956; Luban-Plozza 1959). Personal appearance, particularly of the face and teeth, probably never played such an important role in a person's self-confidence and esteem as it does today. Most people fear that bad teeth make them look older, less fit and generally the worse for wear. They thus tend to attach more value to their anterior teeth than to the less visible premolars and molars, despite the important masticatory function of the latter. This is, however, a relative aspect, and it can be said that people assess in general their teeth very highly. Yet when we consider the lack of care and self-discipline in individual dental health, the disregard of the most elementary preventive measures, it must be concluded that this constitutes a psychological problem. Great progress has nevertheless already been achieved over the years by dint of prophylactic dental treatment. This can be maintained and even improved only if individual responsibility for personal dental hygiene is encouraged and not endangered by undue importance being attached to charges and insurance (Marthaler 1978).

5.3 Going to the Dentist

Going to the dental surgeon is often a stressful event associated with anticipatory anxiety, a general feeling of oppression, and autonomic dystonia

(Kielholz 1974; Pöldinger and Labhardt 1988). Despite the extremely effective pain killing techniques of our time (from local anesthetics and analgesics, to sedation) dental treatment is still experienced by certain patients as painful, even aggressive (Radanov 1983).

It should also be realized that patients often make their way to the dentist with certain feelings of guilt since they assume they are themselves largely responsible for their complaint. Anxiety and feelings of guilt are probably the most important factors which cause the patient to neglect having regular dental inspections.

Anxiety prior to dental treatment is found in all strata of society and in all age groups. It is often based on old ideas of the dentist being a kind of bogey-man with instruments of torture and partly on traumatic experiences in childhood. These conceptions are reinforced by fears from the collective unconscious, which can be proved psychologically, and which persist despite the development of modern sophisticated dental methods and techniques for alleviating pain. These fears have remained the subject of caricatures and comic strips, whose odd descriptions of mishandled patients unhappily strengthen such apprehensions instead of helping to eliminate them.

The modern dentist's chair, in which the patient can be tilted into any desired position, makes for a technically optimal treatment, but for some people it constitutes also a particular stress situation. The close physical proximity of the surgeon, along with difficulties in verbal communication imposed by the instruments, are further factors that in some patients elicit feelings of defencelessness and helplessness. This anxiety may manifest itself in various reactions, for example, in fleeing from treatment or putting it off, aggression, defence, using force and even biting. It may have a crippling effect on certain psychic functions in the form of stupor, which is evidenced by stiffening and spasm, making it impossible for the patient to relax. This necessitates investigation into the underlying causes.

Patients strongly influenced by this background of anxiety find the situation all the more oppressive if they feel alone. Being alone in the waiting room or in the company of fellow sufferers tending to potentiate their anxiety, together with their nervous inability to find a distraction, increases the feeling of helplessness and hopelessness. This initial situation should be taken into account in the interests of patient and dentist alike in organizing the practice and in particular in establishing personal contact (Elhardt 1962; Manné 1970).

5.4 The Dentist-Patient Relationship

As far back as the sixteenth century, Michel de Montaigne expressed his psychological analysis of pain along the following lines: man does not suffer so much by what happens to him as by the way in which he accepts it. This is also true of dental treatment. The first contact and talk between dentist and patient may prove decisive for the later behaviour of the patient and the course of the treatment. The dentist must be aware from the outset that modern psychology no longer views the fear in the forefront as pathological malfunction but rather as a normal, healthy reaction in the form of a warning system. He should accordingly bring the patient to recognize his fear for what it is, to live with it and master it. A dentist must also realize that patients today want to be appreciated as partners, especially as they no longer consider themselves as medical or dental illiterates. Sometimes to their advantage, sometimes to their disadvantage, they are often considerably informed by the mass media and expect perfect dental techniques in the same measure as they do human understanding for their needs and requirements – including financial aspects. They have become more critical, alert, and – thanks to information given over the years – more health and dental conscious. They are consequently more susceptible to motivation by an understanding verbal approach and being won over to a long-term partnership.

On entering the surgery the patient automatically expects the dentist to give him the reassurance and support that will help him overcome his anxious expectations. He feels somewhat lost in this environment permeated by hygienic odours and glistening with technical perfection. This can be countered at an early stage by an understanding receptionist or assistant. If a dentist shows the necessary empathy from the very beginning, listens quietly to the patient and then helps to allay his anxiety, he will win the all-important confidence of the patient. The time thus expended will be rewarded by a more relaxed patient who is easier to treat. In order to establish this empathy it is very helpful to pay attention to such everyday features as the tone of a patient's voice, the manner in which he presents himself or the state of his hands, e.g. whether they are dry or cold and wet. If considerable clinical reconstruction is necessary it is advisable to draft out a plan of the treatment. In doing so, one should take into account the patient's social status, emotional condition, his own particular requirements and financial situation (Joris; Schärer).

Finally, the influence of the dentist's own state of health on the success of the treatment should not be underestimated.

5.5 Psychological Aspects During Treatment

Dental treatment takes place in an area that is particularly sensitive to emotional influences. The inevitable, face to face proximity can evoke in sensitive persons the impression that their conscience is being laid bare, their most intimate feelings being probed to the very bedrock of their personality. The patient frequently anticipates reproach owing to his neglect of dental care and the accompanying warning. This makes him feel like a scolded child caught in some misdemeanour and provokes his opposition (Luban-Plozza 1969). Owing to lack of knowledge of the many different psychological, psychosomatic and sociomedical problems involved, all too many dentists desperately resort to conventional authoritarian and even repressive methods; they take refuge behind the myth of salutary infallibility surrounding the white coat. If, however, psychological and psychotherapeutic experience still fails to produce the desired result, the use of a psychotropic drug is also indicated. In view of the growing number of drug addicts, this can be problematical and should be resorted to only after careful consultation with the patient's family doctor or a relevant specialist (Kielholz 1974).

5.6 The Various Groups of Patients

Thanks to a wider appreciation of dental problems on the one hand and the efforts of dentists towards better mutual understanding on the other, most patients are happily in a position to master their anxiety quite well by themselves. Certain groups of patients, however, place increased demands on the dentist's psychological ability. To these belong children, who tend to be labile and emotionally oversensitive during their development, and particularly neurotic patients with their unconscious fears and conflicts that have not been worked through (Elhardt). Another group is made up of old and incapacitated patients, whose social and health problems present the dentist with additional commitments.

Dental Health Care in Children

This is ideally commenced as early as pregnancy by informing the parents on means of preventing dental trouble. Their attitude to dental problems will largely shape the child's behaviour in this direction. Childhood experience in the surgery contributes greatly either to later fears and opposition or to insight and understanding (Schäfer et al. 1974).

Owing to the increased number and severity of developmental disorders in young people, psychological and social problems must be accorded more attention than was previously the case in present-day dental care of this group. We shall accordingly have to reckon with more children and adolescents among our patients who both physically and emotionally have less resistance to stressful situations and increasingly manifest depressive behaviour.

It should be generally accepted that dental treatment invariably constitutes a stress for children, and its intensity depends on the excitability of the young patient. Children tend to project their personal problems and fears into the treatment. For this reason it is important to know something about their family milieu. They experience dental treatment as a conflict situation far more than adults do; it is a situation into which they are forced against their will and cannot resist without being punished. Children see themselves confronted by a problem to which there is no prospect of a satisfactory solution (May and Squazorni).

Even the waiting room is hardly suited to their age and emotional condition with respect to reading matter and toys for diverting their fears and allowing them to relax.

Of particular importance is the behaviour of the parents accompanying the child. It is by no means infrequent for them to experience their own residual fears along with those of their children. They are thus unable to comfort the child or distract him and prevent such childlike manifestations as a firm refusal to enter the surgery or even open his mouth once he has done so, not to speak of the occasional screaming and kicking. The reasons for such behaviour, which may arise even in the absence of previous experience of dental treatment, have not been thoroughly explained. It has been established that girls are generally more nervous than boys (Luban-Plozza 1969).

When treatment is imminent, the general bearing of those accompanying the child, whether parents, siblings or friends, acquires decisive significance. Anxious behaviour, lack of composure, or faulty attitudes on their part can become models for 'social imitation' and trigger off anxiety even if the child has had no traumatic experience of his own. Some of these people prove to be more of a liability than an asset, even though they act with the best of intentions.

Experience has shown that later dental treatment is made considerably easier if one of the parents brings the child to the practice for some reason other than having treatment. This will enable it to become familiar with the surroundings without any painful associations.

The dentist unfamiliar with treating children has sometimes a tendency either to adopt an authoritarian manner or resort to the use of sedatives or even general anesthesia. But this will not solve the problem of anxiety. There is, by the way, nothing against the child bringing along a teddybear or favourite doll if this is of help. The main thing is that the visit should follow a set but friendly pattern from beginning to end.

By splitting up the treatment into individual sections, always performed in the same sequence and explained to the child in simple language, our very young patients are put more at their ease since they are then confronted only with familiar procedures. With short pauses (mouth rinses, refilling the glass) we can to some extent meet their urge to move. The aim afterwards is ideally to create some form of success experience, no matter how modest, at the end of each visit in order to build up their self-confidence (Loch).

Nervousness, uncertainty and hectic conditions make children restless, anxious and aggressive. A friendly, self-assured manner with appropriate facial expression and voice control are essential for the success of the treatment. As a patient, the child must feel the centre of all our endeavours and the most important person to talk to.

In schools and homes, the presence of several children together in the same consulting room has proved to be of great advantage. The mutual help and encouragement afforded improves understanding of the course of the treatment and facilitates tolerance towards objects usually generating anxiety, such as dental drills and injection needles. An important condition is that both examination and treatment are carried out in the same sequence for all in order to avoid any hint of confusion or insecurity. Teamwork is of particular importance for instruction, motivation and practice in the prophylactic sector.

In orthodontic treatment the child is subjected to far more emotional stress than in, say, preventive dentistry or restorations; the dental anomaly itself or the wearing of an orthodontic appliance not infrequently gives rise to feelings of inferiority. The proven psychosomatic aspects involved in orthodontics have been neglected even up to the present by virtue of treatment based largely on technical assessment. Even in children there is background to dental malformations of unresolved personal conflict and difficulty in social adaptation as well as of heriditary factors. These psychosocial factors have been shown to have their origins in disturbed relationships between mother and child in earlier life. They must therefore be given consideration within the scope of putting in order masticatory and speech functions of such a young person still in the stage of development.

Disorders in the audiovocal sphere resulting from neuromuscular dysfunction demand particular human and psychological abilities. Yet they can be overcome only in teamwork between logopedic specialists, physiotherapists, orthodontists, parents – and the children themselves (Assal; Loebell).

Prophylaxis in Adolescence

Children learn correct care of their teeth and sensible eating habits very much in the same way that they learn reading, writing and arithmetic (Magri). The motory and mental habituation must adapt to that needed for oral hygiene. This is achieved by dint of information, training and repeated motivation, so that one could almost speak of a programming process.

The 'dental consciousness' developing within the scope of collective and individual prophylaxis not only promotes the self-responsibility essential to oral health when schooldays are over, but also largely determines the attitude of the individual to dentistry.

It is thus very important that instruction in oral prophylaxis is given without moral undertones. Should the ever possible caries develop despite good care, feelings of guilt might then arise with the resulting feedback of fear of the treatment that became necessary after all.

Rather than lay too much emphasis on the complete absence of caries, the target of prophylactic instruction should be sensible care of the teeth and a positive attitude towards dentistry, thus contributing to reducing anxiety in future treatment.

In addition to the example set by the family and influence exerted by the school medical service it is primarily the attitude of the teacher which decides whether or not pupils continue to exercise preventive measures and have regular check-ups after leaving school. If the teachers themselves are enthusiastic about such measures, habits acquired by the pupils in the interest of oral hygiene have a good chance of becoming firmly entrenched 'dental consciousness'.

The efforts required later in preparing for a profession or trade, often involving changes of address, the loosening of family ties and personality developments while growing up, are a few of the factors having negative influence on oral hygiene till the youngsters realize their responsibility.

Young people with congenital mental or physical handicaps, those with learning disabilities, drug addicts, and juvenile delinquents have particular problems in oral prophylaxis. Experience shows, however, that collective prevention is possible even in homes for the disabled if there is a positive attitude on the part of the staff and a dentist to carry out inspections. These young people need very kind, but firm guidance on the responsibility and activities that can be expected of them.

In the remaining groups there are complex emotional states generally indicating a weakening of the personality. This may be reflected outwardly as passivity, aggressivity, or awkwardness. Here, more than anywhere else it is not enough merely to explain, but very important to listen, and, without sparking off a crisis, get to know what led to such states.

The following are a few basic rules for successful prophylaxis with a positive bias:

- Avoid any reproach, so as not to awake feelings of guilt.
- Make inspections appear as help and not as a test.
- First mention any success before correcting.
- Give information in digestible portions.
- Discuss cases with the team.

Difficult Patients

There are the restless patients who go from dentist to dentist, continually on the look-out for a confidant; and there are those who are demanding and stubbornly insist on a specific treatment. But there are those who constitute particular problems. These are characterized by neurotic anxiety and may be classified under four main types of personality structure, namely, hysterical, compulsive, depressive and schizoid. The problem may assume the form of increased susceptibility to anxiety or that which is masked and not easily recognizable. It may even become manifest in the form of attacks, bouts of unconsciousness and vomiting. They are the outcome of previous experiences and influences, particularly those of early childhood, and simple persuasion or coaxing is generally useless in neutralizing them. Knowledge of the background to such behaviour can in itself lead to a tolerable dentist-patient relationship and make treatment possible. In most of these more serious cases, however, specialist aid is indicated (Elhardt).

Patients with a predominantly hysterical structure present most of acute problems. Their anxiety is easily converted into such physical manifestations as bouts of various kinds and unconsciousness. Their heightened state of suggestibility renders them amenable to psychiatric help. They are relatively easily influenced by the calm, objective and benevolent attitude of the dentist. The effect can be increased if this attitude assumes a rather pampering character, exhibiting warmth of feeling mixed with heartiness and humour.

Patients with compulsive neuroses are mostly tensed, inhibited and full of doubts and hesitation. Their lack of decision delays their visit to the dentist. Marked compulsive symptoms such as incessant washing, cleaning and rinsing may hinder dental work, which is frequently only possible after psychotherapy. The anxiety of these patients is often transferred to purely physical manifestations in the form of pallor and rapid heart beats. In this case a thorough cardiovascular check-up is indicated (Elhardt).

Patients with depressive personality structures comply readily with the dentist's instructions, but this should in no way deceive us about their limited psychic resistance to stressful situations. For them the teeth have a greater symbolic value. This is why they take the loss of a tooth, or damage to it, more tragically than other patients. It is advisable to make careful enquiries into their reactions during previous surgery, dental or otherwise, in order to plan the treatment. It is most important to approach these patients as a person and not just as a 'case'.

Schizoid patients. Owing to disturbances in early emotional development, a relationship to their environment is either lacking or at the most unsatisfactory. Their emotional 'undernourishment' in early childhood produces a primary distrust that may lead to a querulous attitude, hypochondria, enmity and even provocations against the dentist. They constitute the most stressful situation in dental work from a human point of view. Yet should the dentist weather this affective situation by dint of his patience, benevolence and objectivity, his empathy and psychological prowess will be rewarded by gaining the patient's confidence and trust (Elhardt).

Prisoners undergoing a sentence are to be counted among the more difficult patients owing to their particular situation implicating anomalies of character, as well as those of emotional and social conditions. Studies have revealed heightened psychological problems. Convicts exhibit in particular a marked indifference for oral hygiene, little readiness to cooperate in essential matters of prophylaxis and an increased desire for sweetmeats – mainly by drug addicts deprived of their 'stuff'.

A dental appointment does not just constitute an opportunity for convicts to establish contact with the world outside the prison walls; in giving them personal attention and allowing them to feel that it is worthwhile to keep their teeth in good condition like any other citizen, they will be helped to win back gradually their lost self-esteem. The dentist can thus contribute to re-establishing their emotional equilibrium in the general sense of a resocialization process.

There are also very difficult patients who do not fit into any of these groups. These are mostly emotionally labile or sick people who frequently pose insurmountable problems. When neurological or psychiatric symptoms are present, close cooperation with a psychotherapist is indispensable (Reisner). There are also a considerable number of patients who cannot be moved about freely owing to age or incapacity and require special methods of treatment. The handicap may assume many forms, such as physical disability, retarded mental development, congenital defects, metabolic and systemic disorders, spastic states, autism, blindness, deafness, hemophilia and neoplasia. Dental treatment of these patients requires quite special aptitudes, in the first place that of being able to exert a calming influence on them, while in certain cases some modification of the usual practices of preventive and restorative dentistry is necessary. Their needs and requirements are unfortunately often neglected, particularly when they live in homes or are otherwise restricted. Some countries already have excellent schemes in progress whereby such handicapped citizens receive dental treatment within the scope of a team comprised of doctors, relatives, social workers and teachers (Zimmermann).

5.7 Psychogenic Influences in the Maxillofacial Region

Psychosomatic factors play an important role in functional disorders of the stomatognathic system. Studies on the personality structures of patients suffering from myoarthropathy show correlations between the primary somatic disorder and general psychosomatic disturbances. For this reason, relevant psychohygienic and psychotherapeutic aspects should be accorded more attention (Bruch). Similar conclusions were drawn from observations in masticatory dysfunction, particularly when it related to temporomandibular articulation, in 'dentofacial orthopedics', in prosthetic reconstruction and in orthodontic procedures (Weinberg; Zarb and Carlsson).

Different forms of pain in the head and face are often sequelae of true depression and neurotic reactions to postural defects involving the cervical part of the spine, emotional stress playing a major role (Baumann; Drommer). Most of these causes may also be attributed, along with other factors, to inflammatory changes in oral mucosa and in the periodontal region, as well as to dermatoses, burning sensations in the tongue and even herpes zoster (Cooper; Perko; Wespi).

A special problem is constituted by drug abuse and alcoholism, both in respect to changes of psychogenic origin in the mouth and from the treatment angle. Possible drug-induced changes in metabolism and behaviour call for joint efforts with a psychotherapist (Gerlach and Wolters). Generally speaking, the dentist's awareness of the neurovegetative or psychological background of such organic or functional disorders will keep him from going ahead with pointless, purely somatic treatment. He can help the patient only if he recognizes the psychic, anatomical and pathological interrelationships present and works together with the appropriate specialists (Assal).

5.8 Loss of Teeth

Although there is certain evidence that loss of teeth is on the decline – thanks to more enlightened attitudes – extraction is still part of routine practice. It would thus be wrong to ignore the importance of emotional reactions arising from loss of teeth and the interpersonal relationships, including even marriage, than can be endangered. For these reasons alone, it should be endeavoured to restore the aesthetic aspect given by the teeth as quickly as possible.

Owing to the primal symbolism of these parts of the body, the extraction of a tooth or the cutting of the hair is often unconsciously equated with castration or emasculation. Hence, between the loss of a single molar and the loss of all the teeth is a whole range of not only organic and functional impairments but also of psychic reactions to these different contingencies.

The loss of the anterior teeth is experienced as a narcissistic trauma since it is conspicuous and impairs speech. Even the loss of part of a crown can give the impression of neglect and bring the impression of falling low in the esteem of others. In an attempt to prevent the defect from being seen, facial expressions are modified. Great importance is attached to regaining a 'radiant smile', while less importance is attached to putting in order the masticatory function in less conspicuous areas. The way in which a person copes with the loss of teeth depends on the patient's age, sex, social position, psychic constitution and disposition, current circumstances and attitude to his environment. The sudden confrontation of loss of the teeth is fraught with tragic irony since their value appears to be appreciated only after they have been lost. This may cause feelings of remorse, guilt and inferiority. Relatively young people such as adolescents and recruits can usually cope more easily and quickly with the loss of the teeth and master any emotional stress that may arise. The dynamic attitude peculiar to their age, and successes in this period of life, are strongly in their favour. The total loss of teeth in later life is an event that usually gives rise to an anxiety state, sudden shock, or feelings of anguish and hopelessness with a depressive character. The degree and extent to which this occurs will largely depend on individual emotional and mental attitudes. Total extraction is sometimes equated by the patient with decreasing vitality and increasing infirmity, women in menopause being particularly sensitive in this respect. There are other patients, however, who think of it simply as the will of nature and accept it with humility and resignation (Dolder).

5.9 The Dental Prosthesis

Improvements in medical and social care of aging people has led to an increase in the number of patients who require dental prostheses not only for practical reasons involved in eating but also with a view to improving their emotional well-being. What has already been discussed in the section dealing with the different groups of patients also needs to be taken into account here, experience having shown that these patients set more store by good cosmetic results than they do by technical and functional perfection. Yet there is always the problem here of matching the patient's hopes and subjective requirements – 'at last white teeth in an aging mouth' – with objective possibilities and his financial situation. In the case of partial dentures, consideration must be given to the amount of insight the patient has into the matter of oral hygiene and his dexterity in handling such prostheses. This will largely determine the type of denture prescribed (Aeschenbacher and Brunner).

It is a popular fallacy that full dentures have the sole purpose of restoring masticatory function in a purely technical sense; on the contrary, they must be seen in the broader context of physical and psychic factors. Psychosomatic and geriatric problems involved in installing dentures are becoming more frequent in reconstructive dentistry. Such problems are naturally related, on the one hand, to the natural process of aging in the stomatognathic system and, on the other, to less easily understood complaints of psychogenic origin. The latter range from abnormal personality developments to schizophrenia. This may give rise to difficulties in the 'incorporation' of the prosthesis, that is to say the complete adaptation of the patient to it. These difficulties, which can lead to intolerance of the denture, may take the form of burning sensations on the lips and gums, trouble in swallowing, dryness, alteration of taste, a feeling of trauma and impairment of the motoricity of the accessory masseter muscles (Körber; Mellgren; Müller-Fahlbusch).

5.10 Conclusions

Today's dentist is increasingly being confronted with psychological, psychosomatic and social problems. These are frequently the effects of our present-day modes of life and work which are sometimes hardly conducive to satisfactory emotional equilibrium and personality development. These problems make many demands on doctors and dentists alike with respect to plain human understanding and applied psychology. It is clear that more training facilities must be provided in order to develop those abilities that we consider so important in therapy. This would also enable the dentist to work together in special cases with psychotherapists, psychologists, pediatricians or speech therapists. Education and training unfortunately continue to neglect the aspect of character and emotional understanding necessary for this type of work. The psychologically orientated postgraduate training offered by Balint groups would also give the dentist a better understanding of his own personality and thus enable him to recognize the psychosomatic correlations involved in illness. This would make a valuable contribution to the rehumanization of all medical and surgical professions and fill in the gaps left by an all too specialist-minded, technically orientated training (Leatherman).

6 The Psychosomatic Patient After Onset of Middle Age

Bodily health and the sense of well-being relate largely to the success of our efforts in developing our personality and in giving meaning to our lives.

In speaking of 'psychosomatics in older people', we are not referring in this sense to a specific clinical profile. What we understand by the term is rather the many different forms by which physical illness may be manifested in older people in view of the situational crises that aging brings with it.

At the same time, by psychosomatic medicine we invariably mean a psychosomatic approach adopted by the physician in dealing with the patient. This infers that 'psychosomatics in older people' concerns the help that can be given to people who have crossed the threshold between the end of physical development and the beginning of aging.

Petzold (1988b) uses one of Brecht's stories to illustrate the challenges and limitations of old age:

> You remember her perhaps: she was 72 years old as grandfather died. He had a small factory and she kept house for him. Grandmother also looked after the workers and five of the seven children she had borne. She was a small, skinny woman with darting, lizard-like eyes but slow of speech. Of her children, two girls had gone to America, two boys had also left the region, and only the youngest lived in the same town. He was a printer and had far too big a family for his three-room apartment. After the death of their father, the children wrote to one another about the problem of what was to be done about their mother. One wanted to offer her a place to live. The printer wanted to move to her with his family into the large house, but she rejected all their suggestions. The children gave in and sent her a little money each month for her keep. They consoled themselves with the thought that at least the printer lived in the same town. He kept the others informed about their mother in his letters, and was disappointed from the outset that he could not move into the house. Sometimes she visited him and even helped his wife with the preserves. On occasions, she made disparaging remarks about the cramped conditions. (This he reported with an exclamation mark). He wrote that she now often went to the cinema. This was not very respectable. Even worse, she had taken to frequenting a somewhat disreputable workshop of a much travelled cobbler. It was a meeting place for people of ill repute, out-of-work waitresses, journeymen.

> She dismissed his reproaches with 'they have at least seen something of the world'. And she, who had always cooked for others, began to eat at the inn.

But when Brecht's father came to see her, she set a glass of red wine in front of him and enquired amicably, but not at length, about his family. What interested her most was if the children had cherries to eat. She seemed to set little store on going with him to visit his father's grave. 'I have to go somewhere else', she had said. 'To the cobbler, I'll bet!' opined the printer later. And when she even started to go to the horse races he thought she had completely gone out of her mind and wanted to consult a doctor, but the elder brother was against it.

Brecht commented:

> Strictly speaking, this grandmother lived two lives, one after the other. The first was as a daughter, wife, and mother; the second simply as Mrs B., as an unattached woman without responsibilities, and with modest but adequate means. The first life extended over some six decades, the second over hardly two years.
>
> In this second half she granted herself certain liberties, getting up in summer at three in the morning, for instance, to walk through empty streets. She had the whole town to herself.
>
> She died suddenly on an autumn afternoon in her bedroom, not in bed, but sitting in a wooden chair by the window. Living with her was a crippled girl she had recently taken under her wing. A photograph taken on her deathbed to send to the children, shows her tiny, heavily wrinkled face with its thin-lipped but broad mouth. Much that was in one sense *petite*, but nothing petty. She had savoured long years of near-slavery and short years of freedom, and eaten of the bread of life down to the last crumb.

6.1 Crises in Middle Age

The following sections deal with a few typical critical situations arising after the onset of middle age. We shall examine in particular those connected with decreasing physical capacity, the generation gap, retirement and retrospection.

Decreasing Physical Powers

The approach of middle age inevitably brings with it an awareness of decreasing physical capacity. Sight and hearing become less acute, while shortness of breath when hurrying or climbing stairs is more pronounced than in younger people. Men are often troubled by diminshed potency, while women are affected by menopausal disorders. In short one becomes aware in this phase of life that, although one knows more than before, there are things that one can no longer accomplish so well as in younger years. Setbacks, frustrations and concomitant dysphoric moods could once be compensated by increased endeavour, but during middle age it becomes clear that such capacities for extra effort become progressively less. Since this degenerative process eventually ends in death, anticipation of dying acquires added reality in this phase of life.

Object Loss and the Generation Gap

Aging spells the increasing breakup of relations. Children leave home, friends and relatives die. Mothers in particular often find it difficult to relinquish former duties involving care of their children. Indeed the aging person is in general obliged to cede all kinds of responsibility to which he was formerly accustomed. As von Gebsattel put it, he must die 'life's immanent death'.

Kast is certainly right in stressing that people who feel 'halved' or 'cut in two' after losing a longtime partner are not necessarily immature persons who became involved in a symbiotic relationship. She quotes St Augustine in his despair after the death of his friend:

> For I felt that my soul and his soul were 'one soul in two bodies': and therefore was my life a horror to me, because I would not live halved. (Rhys E, ed. The Confessions of St Augustine [VI] 11, translated by Pusey EB. London: Everyman's Library, 1946).

Kast goes on to say:

> It is part and parcel of life that self-awareness stems mainly from our relationships to others, that we often experience as our 'self' what others have evoked and continue to evoke in us. Our relationship to our own deep, most innermost self is hallmarked by relationships to others, by love in particular.

In this context, Willi thinks of life companionship as having the character of a process directed towards establishing common histories which make their marks and leave their traces. He speaks of the dyadic self,

> . . . the partners no longer perceive and experience independently of one another whole tracts of their self, of their very essence. The violent separation of two lovers can thus give rise to the feeling of being cut in two, as a disruption not only of the relationship but of the partner's own self, which is bled of its strength and structure.

The loss of responsibilities and relationships often leads to isolation and loneliness. This in turn gives rise to a feeling of hopelessness, which creates a climate very favourable to psychosomatic disorders (Engel and Schmale).

Most of our modern forms of society make it difficult for aging people to find new responsibilities. In many cases, their qualities and capacities fail to be appreciated. The aging person suddenly finds himself confronted by a younger generation to which he himself once belonged but which neither understands his sense of values nor he theirs. He is then faced with the most difficult learning process of his life: he must accustom and adapt himself to becoming old. This means that under the present social conditions he must distance himself from the idea that aging is a decline from being worthy to becoming unworthy or the beginning of a deficit process (Oestereich).

The reduced capacity of older people to carry out and expand their range of interest and activities contrasts with their increased experience and individuality. These qualities, however, find little appreciation in a society in which conditions change with increasing rapidity, in which dynamic, elastic and adaptive qualities are the new idols, and in which the addiction for everything *new* gains ground, while respect for experience dwindles. Under such conditions it is only too clear that the younger generation cannot accept its elders.

Old people appear to 'disturb' and have no further claims on life. Grubbe reports on an 80-year-old resident of a home for the elderly, who was formerly a farmer's wife and the mother of 14 children. He asked her why she would not live with her children and she answered: 'One brings up children and then doesn't want to disturb them. One goes one's own way. I've lived, so I've no more claim to anything.'

Retirement

Men in particular are often hard hit by retirement. Schultz speaks of 'retirement bankruptcy', while Jores (1970) used the term 'retirement death' in his investigations carried out on pensioned civil servants in Hamburg. Jores found that the outcome of relatively mild illnesses such as bronchitis was frequently fatal during the first year of retirement. He sees the actual cause of death, however, in the sudden cessation of the daily routine. This 'professional death' is followed by physical death if the pensioner cherishes no hopes of continued fulfillment after ceasing to work.

Particularly endangered are those who have identified themselves too closely with their work and responsibilities. Such an attitude leaves little scope for individual maturation. If they have not developed absorbing interests outside their work, the loss of their role and function can lead to a loss of meaning in life. The building up of a strong 'work ego' after so many years corresponds with the loss of identity at a time when one's working life has finished.

This is even more true of patients whose over-identification with their work constitutes a flight from the emptiness of their lives and has made them addicted to work. Von Gebsattel has given us an impressive description of this type of attitude, which is sometimes equated with that of the 'Don Juans of achievement'. The forcible interruption of this attitude to life can lead to depression, psychosomatic disorders, and, as Jores has stated, to psychosomatic death during the first or second year of retirement.

If frustration and depressive mood is compensated with the aid of increased work and performance, the sudden disappearance of such outlets is inevitably disadvantageous. Even abrupt release from a continuous stress situation is experienced as stress far exceeding that of the protracted situation. The major factor responsible for the collapse of many patients after retirement, however, is doubtless their attitude that the loss of their occupation is associated with all loss of hope for a meaningful life of fulfillment.

At this juncture we should think of the experiences of prisoners-of-war and concentration-camp internees. Many of them, particularly the latter, lived under inhuman conditions. Sometimes only the hope of eventual release and repatriation kept them alive. There are confirmed reports of prisoners living for years in camps, only to die on hearing of the death of their wife or of the total loss of their family. Such tragedies clearly underline the pathogenic character of the collapse of hopes and a loss of purpose.

Retrospection

Growing old demands a certain measure of retrospection. Many aging people find this difficult. After all, age is merciless, we have become what we are, as the poet Charles Péguy expressed it. Looking back on life all too often shows that it was perhaps full of events but did not yield fulfillment and concrete results; it may also reveal that one did not master life but was mastered, that one failed to develop original gifts and even one's own personality.

For this reason, many people avoid the painful confrontation with the life they have lived or failed to live. Repression then holds sway over everyday life. This can manifest itself in resignation, a sort of mental paralysis, or bustling yet aimless activity that Kütemeyer termed 'busy apathy'. This refusal to acknowledge the past may have repercussions in increased anxiety, the feeling not to have lived at all, or in psychosomatic disorders. The feeling 'not to have lived' is held by Fromm (1964) to be at the root of the irrational fear of death.

Aging persons who refuse to compare their endeavours with what they have achieved deceive only themselves in hindering their process of maturation. We feel the tension created between the lifework of a person and the repression accompanying the idea of death. Buf if death cannot be accepted in our everyday life, then neither can older people, who constantly remind us that death will one day overtake us.

6.2 Psychosomatic Disorders

Psychosomatic disorders occur more frequently in the second half of life. There are various reasons for this. On the one hand, emotional strain increases with aging, while abilities decrease; there is at the same time a tendency to compensate inner stress by increased striving for achievement and similar defence mechanisms. On the other hand, older patients tend to develop psychosomatic disorders instead of neurotic and functional symptoms.

Müller (1967) attributes this to the increased potential of 'wear and tear' illness and disability in which the emotional problems can take root. Looked at in this way, psychosomatic disorders in old age would lose their relative specificity; there would be absolutely no point in creating, so to speak, a new, typically psychosomatic clinical profile out of thin air.

It is widely agreed that increasing age is accompanied by a greater frequency of dermatoses. Chronic gastritis, intestinal spasm and constipation are likewise more frequent. Even subjectively, older people devote more time and attention to digestive functions. Busse (quoted from Müller 1967) has interpreted this typical phenomenon of old age as 'oral-anal regression'.

Headache and backache are frequent complaints. The regions of the back are particularly susceptible to psychosomatic disorders. Such patients generally have difficulty in getting to grips with their inner problems. When confronted with frustrating situations and narcissistic ailments they react by directing their aggression inwards, which can have somatic consequences.

Particularly in large cities, many men suffer from functional cardiac disturbances. There is much to be said for the explanation that the hypertension and rheumatic complaints so often encountered in old age are not only 'wear and tear' over the years but also the effects of aggression directed inwards.

Obesity, its occasional association with maturity-onset diabetes, and alcohol abuse form part of the self-destructive pattern of habits shortly before the turning point of life.

Such complaints of predominantly psychic origin have a significant correlation in old age with concealed feelings of anxiety stemming from problems of adaptation. The organic disorders are frequently the expression of a *masked depression*. Even the depression encountered in menopause occurs mostly in the masked form according to Birkmayer.

Engel is of the opinion that many menopausal symptoms already exist before climacterium; although they become more pronounced during menopause, it is by no means their first appearance.

The symptoms existing before the onset of aging thus worsen to a marked extent once this turning point has been passed. This is particularly true of situational crises, and is illustrated by the following observation:

> An elderly widow, who had been living with her son's family for very many years, had gallstones but was largely asymptomatic. This changed after the possibility was discussed of her son having to move to another town for business reasons. Then the gallstones were 'set in motion' and not only resulted in severe colic but also in serious pancreatitis. Both symptoms subsided and resolved with surprising rapidity after the son's plans to move fell through and the *status quo ante* was restored.

The gravest risk during these 'now-or-never' years is a lack of communicative resonance. Marriage partners run the risk of drifting apart after their home has consolidated, when the furniture and fittings are all there, or when they have finally acquired the type of house they had been looking forward to for so long. In such cases there is no longer any relevant goal in sight which can hold them together and structure their lives.

In the lives of estranged couples, mild complaints assume disproportionate importance. It is as if the patients had to become ill in order to enter into closer contact with someone. Thus women tend to suffer frequently from general tiredness – even without iron and calcium deficiency.

If the patient is unable to integrate the process of growing old into his life, it will manifest itself more physically. Should a patient try to elude his regret at encroaching age, deny or repress it, his body will suffer all the more. Such patients exclude themselves as a person from their own body, until it is the body that finally 'speaks'. Their conflict remains anonymous: 'Not I, but my body is ill', they seem to say to their doctor.

The Doctor–Patient Relationship

What is the scope of the physician in the present context? It is well known that medicine has made great contributions to prolonging life. The average expectation of life in 1950 for people living in West Germany was 65 years. In 1971, it was 70 years. In 1950, the number of people over 65 years of age was 94 for every 1,000 of the population. The corresponding figure for 1970 was 128, and 144 in 1980. As Table 8 shows, this development continues; a large proportion of the population lives longer and the number of symptom-free years is increasing.

In actual practice, the patient in this age group is looking for help, and his symptoms lend expression to his hopes and expectations. The doctor then has the difficult task of reconciling the patient with the fact that he is growing older. His words must be thought of as a drug acting against any feeling of hopelessness. Balint established that the doctor constituted the most important medication of all for the patient.

Table 8. Trend of the mean life expectancy of newborn children and 45 year-olds during the last thirty years in the Federal Republic of Germany (D), The United States (USA), Sweden (S), and Japan (J). (After Junge 1988)

Mean life expectancy (years)	Men				Women			
	D	USA	S	J	D	USA	S	J
Newborns								
1950/54	65.2	66.0	70.4	60.5	69.5	71.9	73.2	64.0
1965/69	67.5	66.8	71.8	68.8	73.6	74.1	76.6	74.1
1978	69.2	69.6	72.5	73.2	76.0	77.4	78.9	78.6
1984	71.3	71.1	73.9	74.8	78.1	78.3	80.1	80.7
Change from 1950/54 to 1978 (%)	6.1	5.5	3.0	21.0	9.4	7.6	7.8	22.8
Change from 1978 to 1984 (%)	3.0	2.2	1.9	2.2	2.8	1.2	1.5	2.7
45 year-olds								
1950/54	27.8	26.9	29.8	25.8	30.3	31.3	31.4	28.9
1965/69	27.2	27.0	30.2	28.1	31.9	32.8	33.8	32.2
1978	28.1	28.9	30.4	31.0	33.6	35.2	35.7	35.5
1984	29.2	29.8	31.3	32.1	35.0	35.9	36.6	37.3
Change from 1950/54 to 1978 (%)	1.1	7.4	2.0	20.2	10.9	12.5	13.7	22.8
Change from 1978 to 1984 (%)	3.9	3.1	3.0	3.5	4.2	2.0	2.5	5.1

The doctor must divine and diagnose the patient's prevailing problems from the presenting symptoms and hence interpret the complaint. Adopting a 'humanistic attitude' will also afford an approach to lonely and isolated patients.

In individual cases it may be required of the doctor to assist in working through the task of retrospection dealt with earlier in this chapter. Completion of the picture given by retrospection, the incorporation of the past into the present, can open up a future for the patient. Life in old age then acquires a meaning and can again become active.

It is of great help to the patient to realize in the course of his relationship with the doctor that he can embark on the venerable chapter of his life. The patient needs this help, only if this expression 'venerable', with its intonations of benevolence and respect, seems to be disappearing from current usage. This mood has given rise to a struggle on the part of older people for esteem and consideration, hoping against hope they will not be 'thrown on the scrapheap'.

Mere explanations and advice on the part of the doctor are of little help. The patient's well-being is dependent on his physician allowing him to enter into a working relation, the weighting being evenly distributed over the work itself and the relationship. Only under this condition will the patient gain a feeling of communicative resonance with his doctor and stand a chance of working through and experiencing more hopeful perspectives of old age.

'Doctor's alexithymia' (Luban-Plozza) can thus be dangerous, while a friendly, empathetic approach and a grain of humour can achieve very positive results.

Meerloo aptly summarized the doctor's duty to patients in 'the third age' when he wrote: 'Those who believe they have no future should be referred to the past in order to help them accept the present.'

6.3 Treatment

A thorough physical examination and laboratory tests where indicated are naturally indispensable. This is in no way contrary to our psychosomatic approach or principles.

Some of the basic aspects of treating psychosomatic disorders in patients who have passed the meridian of life have already been explained: the doctor himself acts as an important, perhaps the most important, medication. He must shape a true working relationship with the patient. This alone will be a great help to the patient. The doctor must ask himself – and his patients – a series of questions: In what sort of crisis is the aging patient? How is his everyday life? What has life made him in his old age? A major aim of the therapy is to find something that makes the patient feel useful. And it will not be easy to find an activity matching his energies and abilities. But why should only schoolchildren and students become baby-sitters? Would not grandparents, even great grandparents, be able to replace the fairy-tale record albums to some extent? Would this not provide an emotional boost to the continuity of the generations? It also appears to us that the opportunities of employing older people in some form of social work has not been properly gone into. Encouraging the elderly to use their imagination is also part and parcel of the doctor's task. The 'well-earned rest' often advocated for the aged frequently means, if we are honest, that the young would like to be left in peace.

The doctor should not overlook the possibility of tiredness and exhaustion being the sequelae of loss of purpose and meaning in a person's existence. Few situations are more strenuous than having nothing to do the whole day. We allow ourselves to be too easily deceived by the biological life cycle with its ascending and descending curves. In his mental, spiritual and social essence, man has a continually ascending life curve in that he is to some extent continuously learning new facts, gathering new experience and enters into new chapters of his life with new responsibilities. The elderly are often concerned with questions of a religious or philosophical nature. They are questions that the doctor should not evade.

Suggestions encouraging pleasurable and constructive activities are likewise important. What opportunities are offered by broadcast courses or other facilities for adult education? The patient should also be asked when he last went to a symphony concert, to a theatre or cinema. Occupational and work therapy, clubs for older people and day excursions can only be recommended if they provide new contacts, promote creative ability and heighten self-esteem.

Spa treatments can also have positive effects if they lead to new human contact. They may, however, have the reverse effect and result in depressive reactions if the aging person in question cannot adapt to the general atmosphere and feels even more isolated. Also of importance is the fulfillment, under the given circumstances, of erotic and sexual needs. For contrary to some popular fallacies, the elderly are not asexual.

Well-supervised autogenic training and light physical training place a gradual and careful loading on the autonomic nervous system. Such training has a tendency to reduce vagal excitability. Good results are also obtained by employing the more active types of breathing exercises and functional relaxation.

Mention should also be made at this juncture of the possibilities offered by *family confrontation* in treating psychosomatic disorders after the onset of middle age.

In such confrontations, older people in particular often express a strong need to talk. They appear extremely grateful to be included in the therapeutic process; it is confirmation that an unexpected degree of competence is being ascribed to them for past events. In the presence of the other members of their family, they gradually begin to comprehend certain mistakes and emotional factors underlying their complaints and are able to discuss them together. The object is to clarify the entire family situation and the dynamics involved – in the presence of a doctor who is ready at all times to offer guidance and help but not to pronounce judgement. The more experienced the doctor is in the diagnostic and therapeutic aspects presented by such relationships, the more help will he be able to afford the elderly and their families.

In general, a meaningful treatment will have a twofold aspect: discussion and somatically orientated therapies – either in the form of physical training or medication – complement each other.

Prophylaxis. There is of course no prophylaxis against old age, but it is foreseeable and appropriate preparations can be made in order to prevent or delay some of its worst consequences. In this sense we may speak of a form of prophylaxis, which like all others cannot be begun early enough. Even at the approach of the meridian of life, and before if possible, doctors should make their patients aware of certain potentialities that may stand them in good stead on retirement. When this time arrives, they will then be in the position to say: 'Now at last I can do all the things I hadn't time for while I worked!' Old age can then become a time of true fulfillment.

7 The Cancer Patient with an Unfavourable Prognosis

7.1 Basics

To be afflicted by cancer often means for patient, relatives, and doctor alike a certain involvement in the 'magical' conceptions of the disease. Cancer is experienced as uncanny, even punitive with its pain, and has a lingering nature that appears inevitably to spell death. There is, moreover, a dangerous tendency for the patients to become isolated and even stigmatized rather than to receive due help and attention.

As the incidence of AIDS increases, quite similar reactions are being observed in the active and passive outlooks relating to this disease too.

The emotional and life-threatening situations to which the cancer patient is exposed are a consequence of the large number and variety of possible tumour growths, and of the uncertainty of their course. The patient's own personality also plays an important role, as do the prejudices and faulty behaviour encountered in his or her milieu.

The anxiety of patients revolves round notions of incurability and death. It finds its counterpart in the doctor confronted by his own helplessness, and he too may begin to think about death.

Other sources of anxiety are drastic forms of treatment fraught with risk, the thought of pain and the dread of a long-drawn-out death. In order to counter these fears, cancer patients need relatives, friends and doctors in whom they can confide. Moreover, the doctor also frequently needs explanatory background information in his difficult task of attending to the patient.

Many, perhaps too many, people attend to these patients once they are in hospital. Such a confrontation gives the individual patient the feeling of being alone. Detailed, perhaps whispered discussions at the bedside, which are at the most only partially understood by the patient, merely contribute to the general feeling of insecurity. This may seriously impair later attempts at communication.

It is of course advisable to communicate with the patient 'unarmed'. The patient feels that a doctor or nurse equipped with apparatus such as a sphygmomanometer or injection syringes immediately has the 'advantage', but their increased efficiency is really only of a technical nature. Exaggerated activity or polypharmacy is not in the patient's interest; it merely promotes a 'one-way' doctor-patient relationship.

The tendency to deal with patients at a purely 'technical' level is even more marked when they cannot or will not express themselves. This may be misunderstood; resignation, hopelessness and anxiety are then experienced as rejection with the consequence that such patients receive even less attention and their isolation becomes still greater. An occasional excuse for the failure to establish any working relationship with the patient is the presence of cerebral damage or metastases.

Whether consciously or unconsciously, there frequently appears to be a general tendency to avoid contact with cancer patients. Inner attitudes are unsure, while the doctor takes refuge behind a façade of prudent objectivity. There are sometimes even fears on the part of the doctor to identify himself too closely with the patient and his relatives. The patient's insistent queries regarding the prognosis are registered as a confrontation with his own helplessness and mortality. Another reason for the relative neglect of cancer patients by some hospital staffs is that they can rarely be recorded as a 'clinical success'. In the lay public there is evidence of a deeply rooted fear of infection. Should this attitude to avoid the patient start to spread within his circle of acquaintances, the result may be total social isolation and ostracism.

The physician's preoccupation with a cure may constitute an eventual impediment. Alleviation of the patient's suffering can often be achieved by medication, but one should not forget that another great contribution is the attention given. Nor should we forget that solely our presence at the bedside of the seriously ill and dying patient can have a calming effect. As Milton said, 'They also serve who only stand and wait.'

The mute interaction with the patient, personal help even in small things, simply 'being there', the readiness to continue the partnership as long as it exists are all accorded great value by the patients, who then feel they are at liberty to ask questions whenever they like.

7.2 Informing the Patient of the Diagnosis

Bedside honesty is of general concern here. It is not limited to the doctor in charge of the case but extends to relatives, nursing staff and those acting in a spiritual capacity (Müller 1967).

It is our current practice to try and give patients a clear explanation of their particular illness. This must, however, be done individually with great care and tact, at all times taking into account what the patient really wants to know. When possible, this should be done by the doctor treating the case. The carefully worded explanation should be, of course, relevant to the particular situation, and not be given all at once but in the course of several talks. Even against this, however, objections still come from some quarters.

Yet the possibility of the explanation leading to suicide has been refuted by Fox et al. after their investigations into the suicide rates of cancer patients. Although these rates are higher for tumour patients than for normally healthy populations, they do not correlate with the patients being told of either the diagnosis or the prognosis. It is often put forward that the patients are not even interested in hearing an explanation. This is doubtless true for a few cases only, in which it can be assumed that behind the façade of disinterest even greater anxiety is present.

The explanation is for both doctor and patient a twofold necessity. Firstly, concealment of the diagnosis is tantamount to admitting the total absence of any hope, and the pointlessness of treatment. Secondly, with present-day early diagnostic practices, partnership with the patient is indispensible for treatment involving surgery, radiation and cytostatics.

In a Helsinki cohort of cancer patients receiving psychoanalysis, 40% had been informed immediately of the diagnosis by the doctor in charge of treatment. This circumstance was accepted by all patients, but 17% criticized the sometimes rather sudden manner in which they had been informed without any psychological preparation as tactless (Achté and Vankhonen).

For every patient the diagnosis 'cancer' is traumatic. The consequences may be withdrawal from interpersonal and social relations, regression and passivity. The disease is then experienced as an even greater threat to the ego.

On revealing the diagnosis, the patient must not be left without hope and where possible offered a line of treatment. In so doing, we are promising the patients that they will not be left alone (Koch and Schmelling). Favourable findings should be emphasized in the course of discussion. This strengthens the patient's feeling of self-esteem, a loss of which can impair the mobilization of physical and psychic reserves normally at the patient's disposal. A parallel development to this self-surrender on the part of the patient is resignation on the part of the doctor. Yet even the worst prognosis is not devoid of a spark of hope. Even the most skilled and experienced doctor is unable to say with certainty what the future holds, a fact confirmed by actual experience of the most improbable turns of events despite very unfavourable prognoses.

Yet recourse to 'white lies' or half-truths is only of superficial help to the ailing person, who feels the encroaching weakness 'in his very bones' and experiences an even greater sense of isolation after hopes have been dashed. Patients may even gain the impression that treatment is being given for its own sake, as a matter of form. This naturally increases their anxiety and feeling of despair. Hope can, however, be nurtured by the doctor's readiness to enter into an open and helpful partnership, and even eventually have a favourable effect on the course of the disease.

One example of how conditions of life and the general therapeutic climate can influence the will to live is given by the following history:

A 58-year-old country doctor developed carcinoma of the colon and was operated. After eighteen months there was a recurrence with metastases and ascites. He was aware of the diagnosis but told no one, although his relatives concluded from his behaviour that he knew. He would not go to hospital but let himself be treated by a much younger colleague in a provincial town. His son, who was also a doctor, helped in the treatment but was accepted to a lesser degree than the other physician who was a friend of the patient. The patient repeatedly asserted he would take no analgesics and remained so till his decease. After three years he learned that his daughter-in-law was pregnant and he wanted at all costs to see his grandchild. Despite severe symptoms and intense pain this became his main preoccupation. He made his own decisions regarding the transfusions, plasma infusions and vitamins that were necessary for his survival. In making the puncture for the ascites he guided the cannula of his colleague, saying 'Not there, that's where the tumour masses are, cancer masses in fact. Here's the spot!' He would then make the puncture through the abdominal wall himself. Finally, his hopes of seeing his grandchild were realized when the baby was presented to him one week after being born. When it was baptized, the ailing doctor had a portrait of his deceased father placed in the room so that four generations would be represented. During the following days he made a very cheerful and happy impression, repeatedly spoke of his grandchild and passed away peacefully a week later, some fourteen days after the happy event.

It is generally agreed that the patient should not be informed prematurely, say, during the first consultation. The patient should have already voiced his suspicions (Koch and Schmelling).

E. Kübler-Ross has described five phases through which a patient may pass after being informed of the diagnosis:

1. Refusal to accept the facts of his illness. Takes refuge in isolation.
2. Anger and opposition.
3. Negotiating phase (entreaties to doctors in particular).
4. Depression.
5. Coming to terms with the outlook. Calm and worthy acceptance.

It is important for the doctor to find out which stage of the crisis the patient is passing through. There is no point in breaking the news to patients who are beginning to form some idea of the gravity of their illness but are still in the phase of denial or repudiation. Nevertheless, direct questions should not be evaded. Most patients cannot make much out of the bare medical diagnosis. This must be presented in an easily understandable manner before any valid discussion is possible. These patients are primarily interested in how long they have to live, the consequences the disease will have for their remaining life, the trials to come and the effects of the treatment. The typical question 'Is there any hope for me at all?' is exceedingly difficult to answer with a plain 'yes' or 'no'. It is not really what the patient wants as an answer; the question should be regarded as a signal that he needs a discussion partner.

Giving the true facts is frequently eschewed on the grounds that this is not in the patient's interest. Such a rationalization not infrequently conceals the doctor's fear that confrontation with the diagnosis may lead to a breakdown of the doctor-patient relationship. In this discussion it must be realized that the truth is only relative, that average rates of survival or success are of little significance for the individual patient. Only 'present truths' should be told, and these in careful doses related to the patient's questions.

An inconsiderate disclosure of biopsy findings is quite wrong. It serves only as a means of self-protection for the doctor. When we discover a need on the part of the patient to disavow the malignancy, we should respect it since this is a form of protective mechanism. It must, however, be realized that too strong an involvement in a patient's unrealistic defensive tendencies can lead to a disruption of communication, particularly when both doctor and patient participate jointly in denying the truth. The outcome is the patient's further isolation from doctor and family alike. Baltrusch (1969) therefore recommends helping the patient to face the new realities and providing support in breaking down pathological tendencies of defence and denial.

As their illness progresses, many patients give up this denial and enter into the phase where they quarrel bitterly with their fate. They look for a scapegoat and frequently find one in the form of their doctor, the nursing staff or members of their family. It can be very difficult to look after the patient during this phase.

Sapir's psychological investigations show that therapists frequently accuse the patient's near relatives of not being equal to the tragical nature of the situation. Conversely, in the midst of this anxiety and ignorance, the doctor often becomes the family's scapegoat.

In his role as a partner, the doctor can make it easier for the patient to pass through the phases of opposition, hope and despair. These feelings frequently show an abrupt transition, but they can also exist at the same time, generate considerable insecurity and cause the patient to seek some means of orientation. The experience of a frank partnership, perhaps previously lacking, can constitute a very positive experience. This, together with the dulling of physical sensation, may help the patient to come to terms with impending death.

Death may become a personal problem and not just the end result of an illness. This is illustrated by Rilke in *The Notebook of Malte Laurids Brigge* when he writes:

> 'This excellent Hôtel is very ancient. Even in King Clovis' time people died there in a number of beds. Now they are dying there in five

hundred and fifty-nine beds. Of course the whole business is mechanical. With such an enormous output an individual death is not so thoroughly carried out; but that is, after all, of little consequence. It is quantity that counts. Who cares anything today for a well-finished death? No one. Even wealthy people who could afford this luxury are beginning to be careless and indifferent about the matter. The desire to have a death of one's own is growing more and more rare. In a little while it will be as rare as a life of one's own. Heavens! it is all there. We come and find a life ready for us: we have only to put it on. We go when we wish or when we are compelled to. Above all, no effort. *Voilà votre mort, monsieur*. We die as best we can; we die the death that belongs to the disease from which we suffer (for since we have come to know all diseases, we know, too, that the different lethal endings belong to the diseases and not to the people; and the sick person has, so to speak, nothing to do).'

7.3 Family Participation

The best basis for a true working alliance is constituted by the patient, his or her family and the team of therapists or doctor.

Whoever is in charge of administering treatment must take into account the individual family 'system' and its palette of relationships (Stierlin 1978). What particular significance has the illness for the patient? And for the family? What forces exist while the patient is still alive, at the time of his possible death, and afterwards? Once recognized, such forces are easier to manage. For this reason, the general policy should be to keep the patient's family under observation as well as the patient and consider it is being treated too (Gutter and Luban-Plozza).

There is of course the risk of supplying the near relatives with too much information and the patient with too little. The tendency then is for the relatives to 'go into mourning' prematurely, thus isolating the patient. Ideally, the relatives should be informed to the same degree as the patient if they are to stand by him (Baltrusch 1969).

It is frequently the relatives themselves who ask the doctor to withhold the diagnosis of cancer from the patient. It may then come to situations such as the following, which should at all costs be avoided:

A doctor had taken on the treatment of his mother-in-law. All members of the family refrained from speaking about the true diagnosis, which was breast cancer with metastases. The mother participated in this silence, neither mentioning nor asking about the possibility of metastases. All had the impression that the situation was, under the circumstances, quite peaceful. But the mother was in fact very depressive and spoke practically to no one. This was interpreted as the presence of brain metastases. Three weeks after the death of his mother-in-law, the doctor discovered by accident that the patient had written numerous letters to her deceased husband since, as expressed in the letters, she felt an absolute lack of true communication with her family. She went on to explain in the letters how she wanted to spare the family the sadness and disgrace of cancer in its midst. In this family so intimately connected with medical matters, the patient was quite aware of the consequences of her illness, and the doctor had failed to notice it. Hence, the family's 'discretion' and premature 'mourning' had been both wrong and pointless.

The *double bind* – here the different levels of information of the patient and the rest of the family – makes cooperation with relatives difficult. In such a situation no one can behave in a genuine and natural manner. Everything is clouded in a form of inhibition, while disclosure would be desirable. The family confrontation (see page 202 ff) often proves a valuable aid in opening up the situation.

Attention should be directed to the following points during contact with the patient's family:

1. Avoidance of a *double bind* in the sense of allowing a split level of information to build up within the family.
2. Mobilization of available reserves in the patient's family.
3. The detection of any anticipatory mourning, either on the part of the patient or on that of the family.
4. An offer of continued partnership with the family after the patient's death.

Kübler-Ross pointed out that even members of the patient's family could pass through phases of development similar to those experienced by the patient during the course of the illness. Close relatives frequently suffer from feelings of guilt and a sense of failure. Discussions with the family can afford some relief and prevent such feelings acquiring a chronic nature.

Therapeutically speaking, it is a great blunder to declare the patient a 'psychotherapeutic case' on account of the anomaly presented by his emotional situation and the exceptional strain to which he is subjected. Most patients find personal contact helpful, whereas many react negatively to the word 'psychotherapy' ('I've had more than my fair share of physical illness, now I'm supposed to be mad as well').

It must be admitted, however, that cancer patients with a bad prognosis react not infrequently to this radical event in their lives with such a strong regression of their vital forces that the general picture resembles that of a psychosis. They acquire a completely empty and burnt-out feeling. In such a situation, psychotherapy may be indicated. The form taken by the treatment will be decided by reviewing the entire situation – along the lines of patient-centred therapy – while taking into account the somatopsychic aspects of the specific cancer disease.

The following procedure can be adopted simultaneously as supportive psychotherapy:

1. Working through positive transference in the context of stable object relations.
2. Reassurance.
3. Providing opportunities for verbalization of secondary hypochondriacal delusions and feelings of frustration and aggression.
4. Psychological reinforcement of the somatic treatment plan. This involves resolving any possible conflicts, depression or disturbances arising between patients and the team of therapists.
5. Attempts at third-force therapy, involving irrational, religious and absolute elements.

7.4 Sociopsychosomatic Implications

The significance of psychosocial conflicts for the development of the disease is shown by the following series of reactions, which can have a pathogenic effect on the body: During conflict there is increased stimulation of the hypothalamus and the limbic system, while the sympathetic nervous system manifests heightened activity. At the same time the adrenal cortex and medulla secrete greater amounts of catecholamine and adrenocortical hormone. The increase in catecholamine results in a raised pulse rate, higher blood pressure, increased metabolism and irritability of the myocardium, raised lipid levels, and a higher rate of clotting. Increased secretion of adrenocortical hormone as a sequel to prolonged psychosocial stresses can among other things impair immunological defence mechanisms (Blohmke).

What is of importance here is that the extent to which a person reacts to psychosocial stressors in the manner described depends on the personality structure, i.e. the significance which he attaches to the events in question. According to Blohmke, the stressors involved are social incompatibility, social change, urbanization, change of location, difficulty or dissatisfaction with work, dramatic events, crises, the loss of a close friend or relative, grief, despair, depression and loss of hope. Such stressors can of course precipitate many forms of illness. This has been shown to be particularly the case when patients underwent a change of emotional equilibrium and found their life situation unsatisfactory, threatening, strenuous and conflictual, while being unable to change it. Holmes and Rahe (quoted in Blohmke) tried in a test to determine the degree of strain to which individuals were subjected. Their results showed that even slight life changes correlated with some deterioration of health in 37% of those examined, moderately serious changes were associated with illness in 51% and serious changes in 79% of cases.

These correlations were investigated particularly with respect to cardiac infarction and cancer. If one assumes that a proportion of malignant tumours are triggered by endogenous viruses, lowered immune activity as a sequel to increased adrenocortical function under psychosocial stress could further the growth of malignant cells. The question of whether emotional and psychosocial factors play a role in cancer is very old indeed. Even Hippocrates and Galen considered it. Present-day theories based on the work of Bahnson, Baltrusch et al. (1963, 1964a,b), Grossarth-Maticek, Kissen and Le Shan, Le Shan, and Schmale and Iker, as well as many others, may be summarized according to Dillenz (quoted in Blohmke) as follows. The history of cancer patients reveals particularly frequently:

1. The loss of an earlier, important person of reference.
2. The inability to express hostile feelings and emotions.
3. An abnormally strong emotional attachment to one of the parents.
4. Sexual disturbances.

These results reveal a distinct correlation between psychosocial factors and the occurrence of illness. They confirm the statements of de Boor and Künzler that in the case of some diseases it has not only been possible to prove the significance of psychosomatic factors but also to explain essential points regarding the dynamics involved. These authors go on to say that it should not be concluded from the above that nothing is known about numerous other diseases because their motivating psychosomatic correlations have no etiological significance, but that they have not yet been systematically examined.

8 Aspects of Anxiety

8.1 Basics

In a trend-setting cycle of poems, W.H. Auden dubbed our times 'the age of anxiety'. For many this was exemplified by the fear of the atom bomb, in worldwide extermination, while for others it was the fear of being uprooted or that human values were being degraded. This concept also appeared as trend-setting to doctors as they began to realize that anxiety was becoming the real cause of ever more conspicuous symptoms, and even signs, of illness. The increasing recourse to alcohol and drugs, together with a rise in the suicide rate – particularly in the developed countries – has been interpreted as a sign of growing universal anxiety. Various forms of intimidating circumstances have also been found to exist for those working in our modern, highly specialized industrial society, where the achievement ethic plays such an important role. The vast reconstruction and industrial expansion taking place in the 1950s also had its due component of anxiety. This time, it was not because of the fear of unemployment since at that time labour was in demand; it was more the fear of not being able to 'keep up with the Joneses'. Then, with the onset of the recession came the fear of having to give up much that had been taken for granted, coupled with the threat of unemployment.

Yet it was not only in the practical spheres of social coexistence that anxiety reared its many ugly heads. Philosophy, too, took this problem to task. Existentialism, first developed by Kierkegaard, a Danish pastor, assumed an atheistic character in the work of Sartre and a Christian interpretation in that of Marcel. Heidegger, who rejected the title of existentialist, constituted an erratic block between these two later exponents. Yet all these lines of thought have something basic in common: in his relation to the world, man is an individual dependent on his own resources to overcome all the many anxieties and struggles posed by his life, nursing at the best hopes of better things to come.

The anxiety theme has also left its mark on contemporary art and literature; not only on the works of existentialist philosophers such as Sartre, but also on those of many writers, poets, painters, and sculptors. Yet it was for Kierkegaard to distinguish between object-related fear and free-floating anxiety. This differentiation was adopted by the psychiatrist Jaspers (later philosopher) and used in psychiatry for descriptive purposes. It was, however, justly pointed out by Schulte that this distinction may have become established in the literature but certainly not in practice. This is largely true also for English-speaking countries, but there are slight differences in usage anyway in daily practice.

The German *Angst* is not quite the same as the English 'anxiety' since it embodies more, in that for example, a trace of anguish is present. *Angst*, or the plural *Ängste*, is often heard in daily routine practice when several kinds of fear are meant, for there is no plural form of the German *Furcht* (fear). A similar comprehensive term heard by the English-speaking practitioner is the simple word 'afraid'. Its uses can range from 'I am afraid of failing my family' to 'I am really afraid of that fierce dog'.

However, in English there is considerable overlap between the terms anxiety, fear, and dread. While 'anxiety' tends to refer to a vague feeling of being threatened, 'fear' is more concrete, and 'dread' points in the direction of phobia. This should be borne in mind before reading the following, which is, of necessity, a compromise between German and English usage, though there continues to be feedback in both directions.

Gaupp brought up the question as to whether fear could be relegated to the normopsychological sphere and anxiety to psychopathological phenomena. This question was later taken up by Thiele. Some light may be shed on the problem by making phenomenological distinctions among the different forms of anxiety, i.e. between feelings of anxiety, anxious moods or dysphoria and anxiety affects. According to Rohracher, *feelings* are states which are inseparable from the other things a person is experiencing at the time, but which require an internal or external stimulus. In this respect they resemble drives and occur without involvement of the conscious mind. They are psychic reactions to internal and external stimuli. As opposed to this, Rohracher speaks of *moods* when one feeling persists over a long period or actually dominates the various other feelings present; this then assumes the form of a *basic mental outlook*. Rohracher describes an *anxiety affect* as a feeling that has become so strong that excitation and its attendant physical phenomena are subjectively perceptible. In accordance with this phenomenological differentiation one could say that anxiety feelings and anxiety affects can occur in both normopsychological and psychopathological contexts, while the longer anxious dysphoria is manifested only in a pathological context. This does not, however, answer the question as to whether a sharp distinction can be made in psychopathology between object-related fear and free-floating anxiety, i.e. between fear that is directed intentionally towards an object and anxiety that is not related to an object.

While Binder continues to respect this distinction, Kurt Schneider points out that such a dichotomy creates difficulties since anxiety can, in fact, have an object, as is illustrated by such expressions as 'to be anxious about something'. He thus infers that only fear always has a motive, while anxiety can be either motivated or unmotivated. He also says, however, that unmotivated anxieties cannot be regarded merely as anxieties that have lost their motive, and contends that unmotivated anxiety is a primal feeling of man. Schulte is also against a rigid distinction: in his study of the anxiety syndromes he emphasizes 'anxiety about something' and points out the 'enormous range of possible variations'. Accordingly it would be more correct to speak of anxieties than anxiety.

8.2 Psychopathology of Anxiety Syndromes

The anxious patients consulting us have many and varied presenting symptoms. Sometimes it is the psychopathological symptoms that predominate, at others the psychomotor and autonomic:

1. *Psychopathological symptoms*
   Distressing sensation of constriction;
   feeling of being helplessly at the mercy of some vague menace;
   inner unrest and tension
2. *Psychomotor symptoms*
   Facial expressions indicative of anxiety;
   psychomotor agitation to point of raptus
   or
   psychomotor inhibition to the point of stupor
3. *Autonomic signs and symptoms*
   Dilatation of pupils, tachypnea, insomnia, facial pallor, dryness of mouth, loss of libido and potency, sweating bouts, diarrhea, hypertension, tachycardia, anorexia, hyperglycemia.

The psychopathological symptoms are difficult to describe, and the patients frequently have difficulty in verbalizing them. According to Schulte, the distressing sensation of constriction and the feeling of being at the mercy of some vague threat are particularly characteristic.

Apart from facial expression, there appear to be two possibilities of psychomotor indications of anxiety. One is psychomotor agitation to the point of raptus, while the other is psychomotor inhibition to the point of stupor. These two expressive phenomena enable us to draw certain parallels with behavioural research in animals. An animal that is attacked can react as follows:

1. Flight.
2. Aggression, if flight is impossible.
3. Feign death ('play possum').

In the agitated form to the point of raptus one could see an analogy with aggressive defence, and in inhibition to the point of stupor a parallel with death-feigning. Finally, the autonomic symptoms are of particular importance. They may sometimes be very characteristic when psychopathological symptoms are either absent or cannot be verbalized by the patient. By analogy with 'masked depression', one could speak of 'masked anxiety' in such cases.

8.3 Anxiety Disorders as Defined by International Systems of Classification

Anxiety states constitute a well-known grouping within the World Health Organization's international classification of diseases (ICD), which is at present in its ninth edition. The criteria for these disorders are as follows:

Definition (ICD-9):
Various combinations of physical and mental manifestations of anxiety not attributable to real danger and occurring either in attacks or as a persisting state. The anxiety is usually diffuse and may extend to panic. Other neurotic features such as obsessional or hysterical symptoms may be present but do not dominate the clinical picture.

Anxiety:
- neurosis
- reaction
- state (neurotic)

Panic:
- attack
- disorder
- state

Excludes:
Neurasthenia,
psychophysiological disorders

It was not until the last twenty years that psychiatrists devoted considerable time and effort to the pathological aspects of anxiety, particularly to the panic syndrome. Yet panic attacks had long since been described by Sigmund Freud in his work on compulsion and phobia.

In the Diagnostic and Statistical Manual of Mental Disorders published in 1980 (DSM-III) the term anxiety neurosis of ICD-9 was subdivided into the panic syndrome and the generalized anxiety syndrome. The essential difference between these systems is as follows: ICD-9 leans on aspects connected with the pathogenesis and thus relates also to the Kraepelin model of mental diseases; DSM-III, however, contains only quantifiable diagnoses, their definitions being standardized. This constitutes an undoubted advantage.

In 1987 the revised edition of DSM-III appeared. DSM-III-R definitions are given below for generalized anxiety disorder and panic disorder:

Diagnostic Criteria for Panic Disorder

A. At some time during the disturbance, one or more panic attacks (discrete periods of intense fear or discomfort) have occurred that were (1) unexpected, i.e., did not occur immediately before or on exposure to a situation that almost always caused anxiety, and (2) not triggered by situations in which the person was the focus of others' attention.

B. Either four attacks, as defined in criterion A, have occurred within a four-week period, or one or more attacks have been followed by a period of at least a month of persistent fear of having another attack.

C. At least four of the following symptoms developed during at least one of the attacks:

(1) shortness of breath (dyspnea) or smothering sensations
(2) dizziness, unsteady feelings or faintness
(3) palpitations or accelerated heart rate (tachycardia)
(4) trembling or shaking
(5) sweating
(6) choking
(7) nausea or abdominal distress
(8) depersonalization or derealization
(9) numbness or tingling sensations (paresthesias)
(10) flushes (hot flashes) or chills
(11) chest pain or discomfort
(12) fear of dying
(13) fear of going crazy or of doing something uncontrolled

Note: Attacks involving four or more symptoms are panic attacks; attacks involving fewer than four symptoms are limited symptom attacks (see Agoraphobia without History of Panic Disorder).

D. During at least some of the attacks, at least four of the C symptoms developed suddenly and increased in intensity within ten minutes of the beginning of the first C symptom noticed in the attack.

E. It cannot be established that an organic factor initiated and maintained the disturbance, e.g., amphetamine or caffeine intoxication, hyperthyroidism.

Note: Mitral valve prolapse may be an associated condition, but does not preclude a diagnosis of panic disorder.

Diagnostic Criteria for Generalized Anxiety Disorder (300.02)

A. Unrealistic or excessive anxiety and worry (apprehensive expectation) about two or more life circumstances, e.g., worry about possible misfortune to one's child (who is in no danger) and worry about finances (for no good reason), for a period of six months or longer, during which the person has been bothered more days than not by these concerns. In children and adolescents, this may take the form of anxiety and worry about academic, athletic, and social performance.

B. If another Axis 1 disorder is present, the focus of the anxiety and worry in A is unrelated to it, e.g., the anxiety or worry is not about having a panic attack (as in Panic Disorder), being embarrassed in public (as in Social Phobia), being contaminated (as in Obsessive Compulsive Disorder), or gaining weight (as in Anorexia Nervosa).

C. The disturbance does not occur only during the course of a Mood Disorder or a psychotic disorder.

D. At least 6 of the following 18 symptoms are often present when anxious (do not include symptoms present only during panic attacks):

Motor Tension
(1) trembling, twitching or feeling shaky
(2) muscle tension, aches, or soreness
(3) restlessness
(4) easy fatigability

Autonomic Hyperactivity
(5) shortness of breath or smothering sensations
(6) palpitations or accelerated heart rate (tachycardia)
(7) sweating, or cold clammy hands
(8) dry mouth
(9) dizziness or lightheadedness
(10) nausea, diarrhea, or other abdominal distress
(11) flushes (hot flashes) or chills
(12) frequent urination
(13) trouble swallowing or "lump in throat"

Vigilance and Scanning
(14) feeling keyed up or on edge
(15) exaggerated startle response
(16) difficulty concentrating or 'mind going blank' because of anxiety
(17) trouble falling or staying asleep
(18) irritability

E. It cannot be established that an organic factor initiated and maintained the disturbance, e.g., hyperthyroidism, Caffeine Intoxication.

In splitting up the previous concept of anxiety neurosis, DSM-III-R differentiates between social phobia, simple phobic disorder and generalized anxiety disorder. The history may also include panic disorder with or without agoraphobia or agoraphobia without panic disorder. The remaining categories of anxiety embrace obsessive compulsive disorders and post-traumatic symptoms. Of primary importance in practice is the distinction made between panic syndrome and generalized anxiety syndrome; experience shows that antidepressants are mainly indicated for the former and anxiolytics for the latter.

Since the World Health Organization are working on ICD-10, intended to be valid for 1992, while the American Psychiatric Association have already produced their revised classification DSM-III-R (1987), some degree of reconciliation between the two systems may be expected, but not standardization. German-speaking areas seem to favour ICD-9 in the clinical epidemiological field, while DSM-III-R holds sway in institutions heavily engaged in research.

As far as the practitioner is concerned, some measure of differentiation between various syndromes in necessary where it may have a consequence for the therapy. When someone suffers constantly from symptoms which can in a general way be described as nervousness, tension, and fear, the generalized anxiety syndrome is a possible diagnosis. Although it is basically difficult to distinguish anxiety from depressive mood, it remains to be clarified whether this generalized anxiety syndrome exists independently or is part of a depressive syndrome.

8.4 The Different Origins of Anxiety

If we can leave aside for a moment the distinction made between object-related fear and free-floating anxiety, it will be possible to differentiate the following forms of either fear or anxiety on the basis of their genesis:

1. *Real anxiety* has its origin in a true danger posed by the external world of reality, e.g. the possible hazards of making one's way through unfamiliar, unlit streets near the docks late at night. This is a signal of alarm intended to protect us from danger and there would be little point in trying to treat it.
2. Fear for one's life (*Vitalangst*) stems from within the body and likewise has a signal function; the anxiety a patient has on experiencing a fresh myocardial infarction causes him to keep still and request medical aid. It would be equally pointless to treat this alarm reaction instead of the underlying disease. Anxiety loses its signal function only when its purpose has been fulfilled and the patient is in the coronary care unit; after this point it may have a negative influence on the natural healing

processes and on convalescence. Then, of course, treatment is indicated.

3. *Moral anxiety* arises when we have the inclination to infringe certain precepts that we have been taught to keep, either by example or by prohibition. Although modern educationalists are divided on this issue regarding the value of such anxiety, one must acknowledge that it has led to a great amount of sublimation, upon which not only European culture has been founded but many others too.
4. *Neurotic anxiety* is difficult to separate from moral anxiety but clearly belongs to the pathological sphere even if it is a product of conflicts in early childhood. It stems from real conflicts that have been repressed instead of solved. These repressed conflicts develop into complexes and lead to anxiety. Neurotic anxiety is amenable to treatment, psychotherapy being the most suitable.
5. *Psychotic anxiety* occurs in endogenous depression, schizophrenia or 'organ psychoses'[6]. It must of course be treated, and here psychotropic agents play a major role.
6. *Existential anxiety* derives its name from existentialism and philosophically orientated psychotherapy (logotherapy and Dasein analysis). This relatively recent category comes closest to Kierkegaard's concept of anxiety: a general fear of not being able to master this existence. Psychologically speaking, this would be the fear of self-realization. Riemann has worked out a synthesis in which psychoanalytical and philosophical aspects are summarized. He names four basic forms of anxiety:

   - The fear of self-surrender, experienced as ego loss and dependence.
   - The fear of self-actualization, experienced as insecurity and isolation.
   - The fear of change, experienced as ephemerality and uncertainty.
   - The fear of want, experienced as finality and loss of freedom.

8.5 Coping with Anxiety

Just as there are many different causes of anxiety, there are quite a number of ways in which the mind and body react to it. These are illustrated in Fig. 7.

Normally, anxiety is discharged rationally by solving problems or conflicts. It disappears in many cases once the triggering situation has been clarified at a conscious level and worked through. It can, however, be dealt with by unconscious processes. In such cases, ego defence mechanisms may arise in the form of phobias, for example, so that free-floating anxiety is

[6] By analogy with 'organ neuroses'.

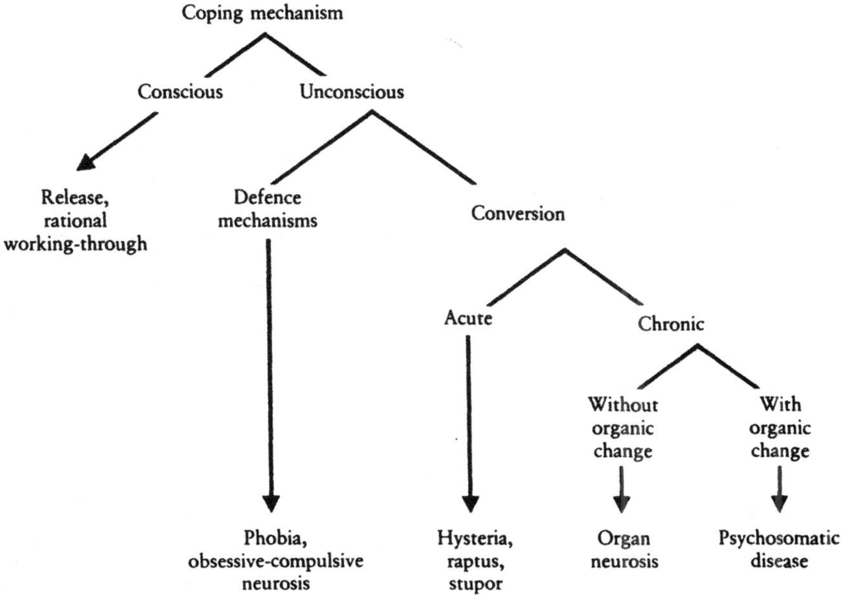

Fig. 7. Reactions to anxiety and mechanisms of coping with it

transformed into exaggerated object-related fears. These may be manifested by a dread of sharp objects, bacteria or confined spaces. Other reactions may assume the form of obsessive-compulsive impulses to count (arithmomania) or to wash (ablutomania). The latter is not primarily the sequel to a dread of dirt or bacteria; it is more of a ritual by which the patient counters the underlying anxiety. If this is stopped, anxiety recurs with fresh intensity.

Anxiety can, however, be converted into physical symptoms, both acute and chronic. The acute symptoms occur mostly via the central nervous system in the form of the classical hysterical conversion disorders, which have now become infrequent. Examples are hysterical paralysis, hysterical blindness and hysterical convulsions. Much more frequent today are the chronic conversion disorders taking place via the autonomic nervous system. If it merely a matter of functional disturbances, we speak of psychosomatic disorders.

By 'psychosomatic disease' we now understand all those psychosomatic correlations in which the emotional problem, primarily anxiety, may lead not only to a functional disturbance but also to an organic defect (see Chapter 2). However, we cannot limit such symptoms to a purely psychosomatic context since they are also seen in endogenous masked depression. The question arises why one person reacts to protracted psychosomatic stress with masked depression and another with a psychosomatic disorder.

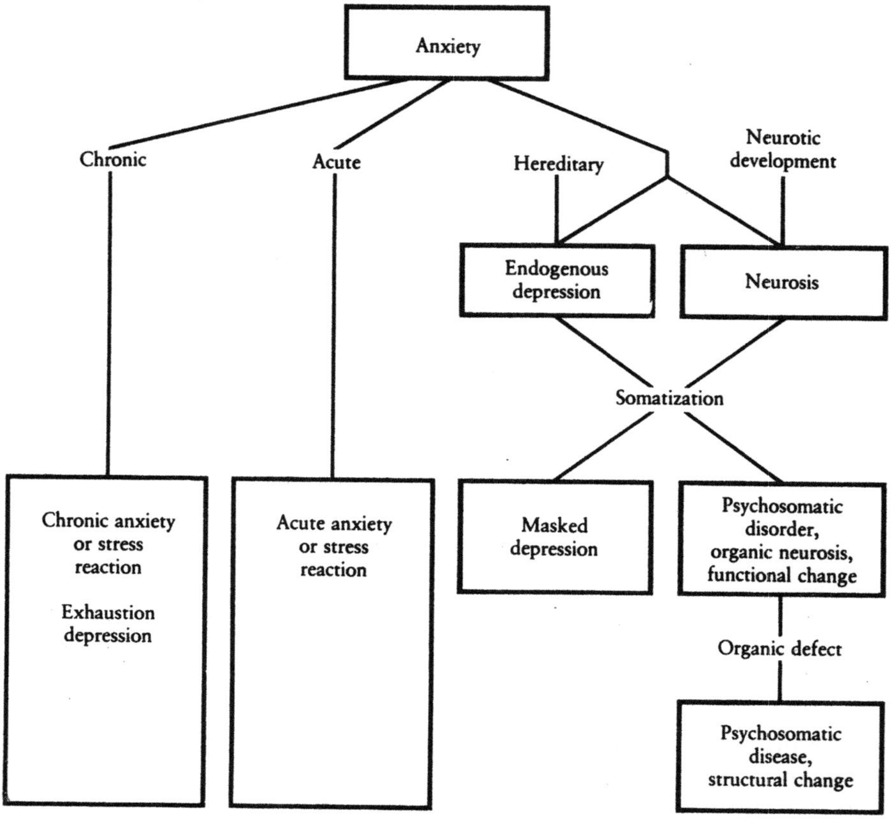

Fig. 8. The relationship of anxiety to psychosomatic and mental illness

Psychosomatic phenomena are thus usually inadequate for differential diagnosis, which can be made only on the basis of psychopathological findings and the course taken by the illness. Fig. 8 sets out several of these theoretical aspects in schematic form.

If we assume that emotional trauma can cause anxiety, this is particularly applicable to the type of personality having a hereditary predisposition to react in a depressive manner. Repression has the same effect, especially in young people with a predisposition for neurosis. Thus, in one case depression may be precipitated, in another a preformed neurotic element resulting in anxiety neurosis. If there is for any reason a predisposition for a given person to somatize psychic processes and energy, the result may be either masked depression or a psychosomatic disorder.

We are much indebted to Strotzka's criticism that this course of events can also ensue despite the absence of triggering factors in the form of either hereditary factors or emotional lability going back to early childhood.

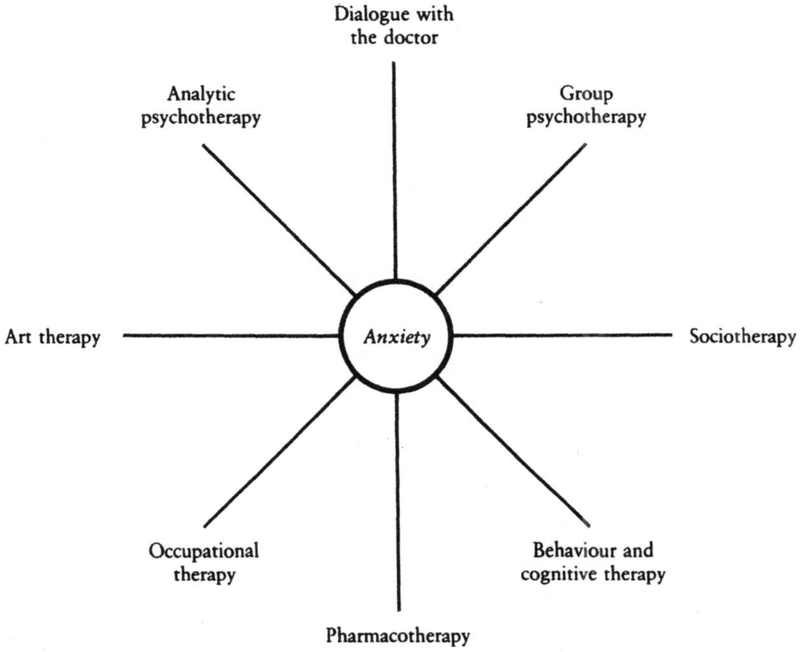

Fig. 9. Treatment of the anxiety syndrome

8.6 Treatment of the Anxiety Syndrome

The most important forms of treatment for the anxiety syndrome are given schematically in Fig. 9.

The dialogue between doctor and patient is the most important part of the treatment since it acts as a catharsis in dispelling anxiety. Moreover, it is during the consultation and subsequent interviews that decisions regarding the various other types of therapy can be made. Today, autogenic training is the first that comes to mind. However, should anxiety occur under specific circumstances and situations, the method of paradoxical intention as devised by Frankl may be employed. Some patients, for example, react to anxiety under certain situations by blushing. Usually, the very thought of blushing suffices to evoke anxiety of the given situation. In using the method of paradoxical intention the patient is trained to prepare himself for the act of blushing, even exaggerate, and in many cases the manifestation then ceases to appear. Treatment employing psychoanalytic psychiatry or nonanalytic techniques in the narrow sense is particularly indicated in neurotic maladjustment and psychosomatic disease. As in the case of the recently developed short-term direct analysis, these procedures should be carried out by specialists only.

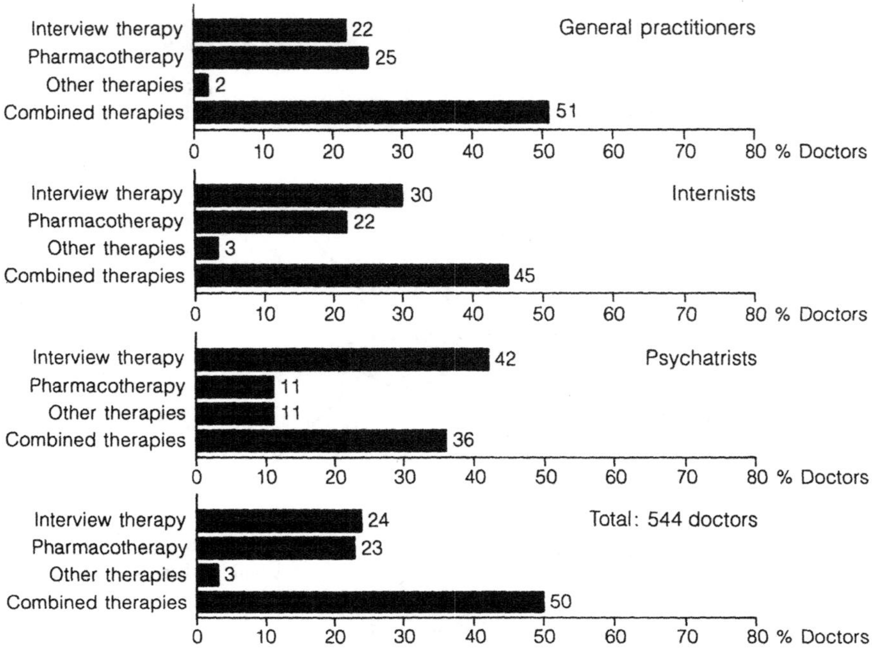

a

	General practitioners	Internists	Psychiatrists	Total: 544 doctors
Tranquilizers (TR)	33%	37%	35%	34%
Antidepressants (AD)	22%	14%	10%	19%
Neuroleptics (NL)	4%	2%	10%	4%
β-blockers (BB)	2%	2%	2.5%	2%
Multiple answers, including combined drug therapy				
TR + AD	16%	18%	7.5%	16%
TR + BB	3%	5%	10%	4%
AD + BB	6%	7%	5%	6%
NL + AD	4%	3%	10%	4%
NL + TR	4%	6%	10%	5.5%
Others	6%	6%	—	5.5%

b

Fig. 10 a,b. Answers to questionnaires sent to general practitioners, internists and psychiatrists

As explained more fully in the chapter on psychosexual disorders, Balint groups are of great help to the general practitioner in learning how to cope with the psychic problems of his patients. This is of course equally true for those involving anxiety. In these sessions, doctors are confronted with their own psychodynamic features, which may under certain circumstances have a negative influence on the efficacy of their treatment and on the validity of their diagnoses. Group psychotherapy has proved valuable in treating states of anxiety of social origin such as loneliness.

Behaviour therapy also has its place in this psychotherapeutic context. As previously explained in this book, a scale of situations triggering off the anxiety must be drawn up for use in the desensitization process. In the sessions that ensue, the stimuli producing the weaker anxiety reactions will be worked on by simultaneous relaxation training. This will be stepped up progressively in further sessions until stronger triggering factors can be worked through without eliciting anxiety.

In addition to physiotherapy and occupational therapy, art therapy can be of great help in combatting the anxiety syndrome. Such creative work not only releases certain affects but also brings them to light. Jacobi showed that it furthered the effectiveness of psychotherapy in a manner similar to dream analysis since pictures too can be interpreted. Finally, no chapter on anxiety would be complete without mentioning drug therapy. Thanks to rapid developments in the field of psychopharmacotherapy, it is now possible to influence the anxiety syndrome in many respects by several different groups of medicaments.

Psychopharmacotherapy

In general practice, anxiety and its somatized symptoms are treated in most cases by pharmacotherapy combined with interview therapy. The latter tends to predominate as sole therapy among psychiatrists only (Fig. 10a). The group of medicaments and combinations most frequently prescribed by general practitioners is shown in Fig. 10b.

Since the anxiety syndrome was split up into generalized anxiety syndrome and panic syndrome, differentiation with regard to pharmacotherapy also arose. While generalized anxiety syndromes respond well to benzodiazepines, the specific treatment for panic syndrome is long-term medication with antidepressants, though attacks can be interrupted with higher doses of benzodiazepine.

9 Masked Depression

By masked depression is meant the existence of depressive states in which psychosomatic symptoms are so marked that it is difficult to recognize the actual psychopathological symptoms.

These in no way constitute a new form of depression. The term is of an explanatory nature. It is a didactic principle bearing in mind the presence of depression in the face of a physical complaint, particularly pain, for which there are neither objective findings nor any somatically orientated treatment to which it will respond. In order to recognize the depression it is advisable to become acquainted with the psychic, psychomotor and psychosomatic elements of the syndrome. These are listed below. When they gain the upper hand, the psychosomatic symptoms dominate the entire picture presented by a masked depression. In old textbooks such symptoms were generally relegated to the footnotes, while today they are considered to be of major importance.

Depressive Syndrome, Symptoms Classified According to Functional Region Affected

Psychic Symptoms
Depressed mood, indecisiveness, inhibition of thought, apathy or inner unrest, anxiety, depressive thought content, loss of feeling, inner emptiness.

Psychomotor Symptoms
Psychomotor inhibition (hypokinesia, hypomimia or amimia, inhibition of vocal expression)
or
psychomotor agitation (physical restlessness, compulsive behaviour, unnecessary activity).

Psychosomatic Symptoms
Loss of vitality (asthenia, staleness);
autonomic disturbances in the narrower sense (dizziness, cardiac arrhythmias, dryness of the mouth, constipation, respiratory complaints);
autonomic disturbances in the wider sense (sleep disturbances, sensations of pain, pressure and cold, loss of appetite, loss of weight, menstrual disorders, impotence).

Important as it is to be on the alert for masked depression, this is not enough by itself; the right questions must be put to the patient in order to establish a diagnosis. For this purpose several questions have been summarized below. The answers to these and further relevant questions should make it possible to determine whether or not endogenous depression is present.

Questions to Reveal Depression

Dejection	Do you feel oppressed and dejected? Do you sometimes want to cry?
Loss of pleasure	Can you still get pleasure out of certain things?
Loss of interest and initiative	Do you show less initiative in your work and spare time than you did a few weeks or months ago? Do you take the same interest as before in daily events, say, in newspapers, on the television or radio? Do your hobbies give you the same pleasure as before?
Failure	Do you consider yourself a failure?
Guilt feelings	Do you often reproach yourself? Do you have feelings of guilt or inferiority?
Pessimism	Do you regard the future more pessimistically than before, and have you sometimes the feeling that everything is pointless?
Brooding	Must you, whether you want to or not, keep thinking about gloomy subjects?
Indecisiveness	Do you find it difficult to make a decision?
Loss of social contact	Have you less contact with your friends and relatives than before, or do you feel neglected by them?
Sleep disturbances	Do you sleep worse than before? Have you difficulties in falling to sleep? Can you sleep through till morning, and do you wake up early?
Loss of appetite	Have you less appetite? Have you lost weight, and do you suffer from constipation?
Loss of libido	Have you sexual difficulties?
Heredity	Were there cases in your family of depression, manic episodes or suicide?
Early phases	Have you had periods of dejection or manic phases earlier in life?
Morning 'low'	When do you feel at your worst? In the morning or in the evening?
Early waking	At what time do you wake up in the morning?

If the general picture is one of endogenous depression in such circumstances, it is evident that we have a case of masked depression to deal with. In the presence of nonendogenous psychoses, e.g. neurotic depression, differential diagnosis for psychosomatic disorders and disease becomes very

Table 9. Stages of exhaustion depression (after Kielholz)

	Hyperaesthetic, asthenic stage	Psychosomatic stage	Depressive stage
Psychic	Irritability, hypersensitivity, sense of failure	Psychosomatic disorders	Depression
Somatic			Exhaustion of the sympathetic, ergotropic, adrenergic system

difficult. Basically, however, it may be assumed that masked depression is primarily a form of endogenous depression that is accompanied by severe psychosomatic symptoms, while psychosomatic disorders and disease tend to be somatized neuroses, which really means somatized anxiety (Pöldinger 1982).

Accurate diagnosis and differential diagnosis are important if only for the reason that masked forms of depression respond very well to antidepressant treatment, particularly when they are of an endogenous character. In the case of nonendogenous masked depression or psychosomatic disorders, combined pharmacotherapy and psychotherapy have proved of great value. Antidepressants are invariably the drug of choice in fact when there is evidence of depression; as opposed to benzodiazepine derivatives, they constitute no danger of habituation or other hazards (Pöldinger 1984).

Among the nonendogenous forms of depression with attendant psychosomatic symptoms should be included exhaustion depression, which was first described by Kielholz. It occurs after periods of prolonged emotional strain lasting a number of months or years. Table 9 illustrates how exhaustion depression first passes through a hyperaesthetic, asthenic stage characterized by irritability, hypersensitivity and reduced functional performance. The second stage sees the development of psychosomatic disorders, in particular autonomic. This corresponds to the old diagnosis of 'neurasthenia' with marked symptoms of fatigue and debility. It is only considerably *later* that the true depressive symptoms appear, either after a period of additional stress or concomitantly with the sudden relief of psychic strain; these symptoms then dominate the third stage and complete the clinical picture of depression.

The possible reactions to emotional strain coupled with anxiety are shown diagrammatically in Fig. 11. If the cause is acute or chronic strain, the patient has either no particular predisposition to the disorder or will show

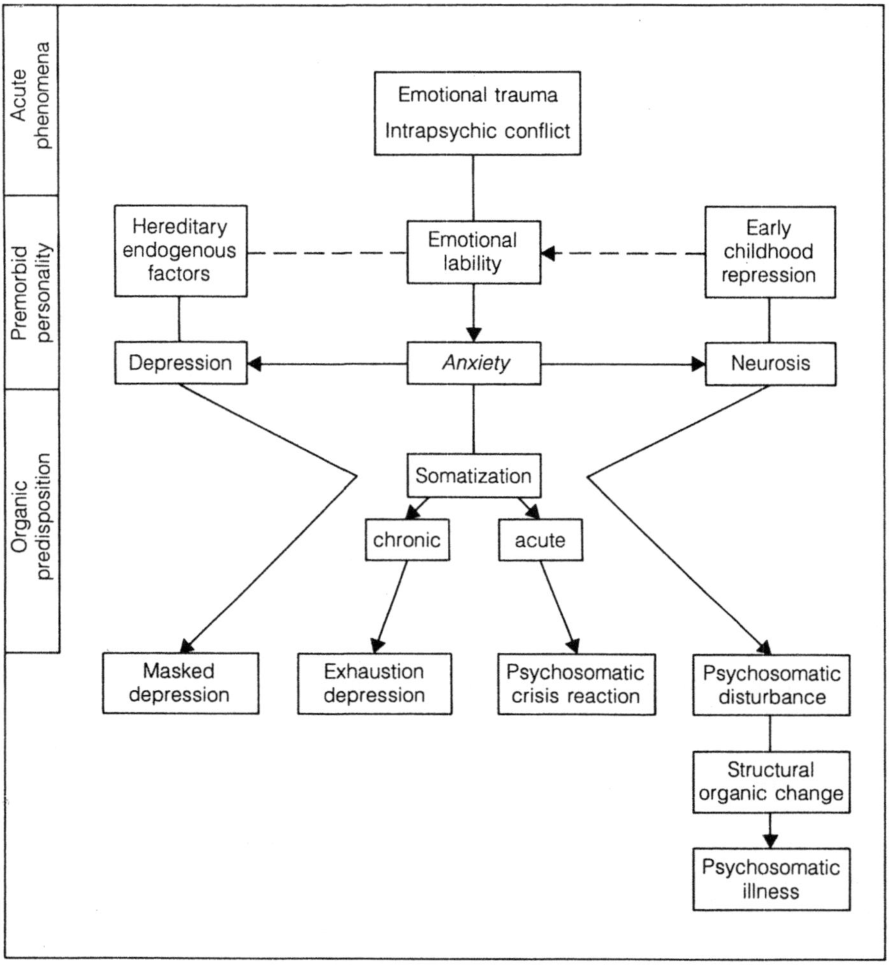

Fig. 11. The most frequent reactions to anxiety

signs of a hereditary, endogenous depression and possibly developmental disorders of early childhood. The reactions to strain should always be taken into account in assessing the case. They may result in exhaustion depression, acute anxiety or stress reactions; an endogenous depression or a neurosis may also arise, depending on the patient's personality. Somatization would indicate the presence of masked depression or a psychosomatic disorder.

10 The Psychosomatic Approach to the Patient

It is important to recognize that somatic medicine and its psychological correlations form an integrated whole. The approach to the patient should be made with a minimum of theory, devoid of any prejudice and without expecting too much at the outset. The over-enthusiastic diagnostician frequently finds this very difficult.

In this vein, Engel (1970) commented: 'Although there are important reasons why a particular disease process must be identified and elucidated as an entity, the ultimate goal must always be to analyse the process as part of the individual's experience of illness.

'This is more in keeping with the obvious clinical fact that the history of a patient is never confined to the neat categories of disease described in our clinical texts. The designation of illnesses or of patients as medical, surgical, orthopedic, psychiatric, etc., reflects administrative convenience and medico-surgical convention, for which the main justification concerns techniques of treatment or examination, not the true condition of the patient.'

Psychosomatic medicine is not confined merely to the patient's illness. Organic lesions, functional disturbances and subjective complaints are seen as intimately bound up with his personality and the background, life and existential crises that have shaped it.

A symptom can be interpreted simply as a signal, but it can also be considered as a type of 'organ language' which reflects the deep-seated tendencies of the personality. Hence the doctor cannot content himself merely with observing and investigating 'neutral signs' in the patient. He must go further and discover the exact significance of the disorder in terms of the factors that shape the illness and govern the patient's life. And this requires empathetic understanding. The doctor-patient encounter is not a simple rational dialogue or a diagnostic interview, nor is it merely an exercise in history-taking. It is rather a joint voyage of discovery into unknown territory. Listening does, of course, play a special role. Yet its essence lies not in keeping quiet or letting the patient talk simply because it does a person good to say what he wants for once, or because every doctor is a kind of father confessor; it lies in giving the patient one's full attention, in being prepared to accept him as he is and take him seriously.

As Meerwein (1960, 1969) put it, 'the doctor needs a "third ear" as it were, with which to receive answers to important questions while the patient is still speaking'.

Psychosomatic medicine is by no means confined to the realms of theory, nor is it simply a humanistic and intellectual approach. It has now largely distanced itself from an etiological approach and evolved into one of relationship. Schüffel (1978, 1988) has described the *psychosomatic approach* simply as a medical attitude.

The term really encompasses an endeavour to rediscover and revalue the original attitude of the physician at a time when highly sophisticated technology and specialization tend to overshadow the relationship between doctor and patient. The task of putting this into practice is of special significance for the family doctor, who is able to take note of the psychosocial situation of his patients at close quarters. This affords him a considerable advantage over his specialist colleagues, particularly over those working in hospitals.

10.1 Problems of the Psychosomatic Approach

The difficulties and forms of resistance confronting psychosomatic medicine are indeed legion. Their causes may be traced in part to the patients, to doctors and to general social conditions.

It has been frequently pointed out that psychosomatic patients are intimately bound up with their ailment, which enables them to establish a kind of labile and painful equilibrium. The physical symptoms afford them emotional release, and the act of transferring some of their mental energy to the physical sphere helps them to get away from their unconscious conflicts.

Efforts to work out what we consider to be better solutions in the course of psychotherapy are frequently met with anxiety and increased defence, which often employ rationalizations of popular concepts of somatic medicine. An example is the ulcer patient who says: 'I've stomach trouble, doctor, not head trouble!' (de Boor 1959).

A mountain farmer once said to us: 'There must be something wrong with my glands, I can't even stand the world going round any more.'

Patients that are so intimately bound up with their symptoms for a long time are not easily convinced by initial attempts to suggest that their complaints may be connected with emotional difficulties. Far more frequently, they wish to hear they have an organic disorder.

Such resistance is particularly marked in patients with painful functional disturbances. Their inner uncertainty and lability, that Seemann aptly referred to as 'falling between two stools', leads them to seek out a doctor who will confirm the presence of a physical complaint and cure them of it.

When one experiences physical pain, the doors of the doctors' consulting rooms and those of the hospitals are open; but often one is not sure – or does not even want to know – what door to knock on when one feels mental pain.

The nonspecialist usually hears only about the unpleasant physical effects and not about the underlying emotions. This becomes particularly apparent when patients complain of tiredness and exhaustion. This they attribute to overwork and exogenous factors even when they exhibit distinct neurotic and depressive traits.

Patients often say they are *tired* when they are in fact meaning something quite different. They may simply need a doctor or be nursing a secret fear of a severe illness such as cancer. Frequently, they want to hear the doctor confirm the relatively harmless complaint of tiredness and have a medicament prescribed. Sometimes this symptom is 'offered' as a cue or signal in order to get into conversation with the doctor.

'Exhausted' patients are often referred to hospital, where there is a place for them and people have the time to take an interest in them, only after numerous medical and paramedical attempts and all kinds of self-medication have been undertaken. This may put an end to the odyssey leading the patient from one doctor to another as far as the local body of the medical profession is concerned, but this is no solution for the physician who must continue to treat the patient.

The inability of many psychosomatic patients to verbalize emotional problems and the tendency to overrate somatic complaints are often the expression of a fear of being stigmatized. The division of disorders into 'respectable' (organic) and 'disrespectable' (mental) is not only common among patients; the doctor too should not be afraid to point out that his diagnosis involves a mental disorder.

Added to this is the frequent difficulty of recognizing the true clinical picture presented by psychosomatic disorders. Unlike neuroses, whose symptoms clearly belong to the emotional sphere, psychosomatic disorders are primarily bound up with organic functions so that their connection with psychic processes are not at first apparent, either to the doctor or to the patient.

In exhausted patients it is particularly important that every effort should be made to establish an accurate somatic and psychic diagnosis before treatment is commenced. The clinical picture of 'asthenia' may mask other conditions such as Addison's disease, hyperthyroidism, malnutrition or incipient cancer. The psychosomatic approach should thus be one of impartiality and constant vigilance for situations calling for emergency treatments, e.g. in the case of a severe asthmatic attack or intestinal hemorrhage in a patient with ulcerative colitis.

This constant readiness to carry out a thorough physical examination and somatic elucidation should in no way prevent us, however, from exerting a psychotherapeutic effect on the patient from the very beginning. This is often very difficult for the general practitioner since his normal medical training has usually not prepared him for such a task. Despite all endeavours and the best of intentions he scarcely knows how to act or what words to use. His dealings with problem patients thus cause him much uneasiness.

The doctor may fear that the patient is taking up too much of his time, or that he is not equal to the challenge of emotional involvement. Perhaps he also feels that if he commits himself too much with such patients he will come across complications in the patient's life that are beyond his ken since they lead him to the very limit of what he had always understood to be his professional duty. It is also often the case that the presenting symptom is not merely the symptom of the individual but a pathological phenomenon of the whole group to which he belongs, mostly the family.

An easier way out, as Bleuler (1961) put it, is to provide a somatic label at all costs; one has only to find a fine-sounding name that gives away as little information as possible and one can bypass the true nature of the emotional disturbances. One of the favourite labels in German-speaking countries was 'autonomic dystonia'. We are well aware today of the havoc that not only physical disorders, but also confused and conflicting emotions can wreak on autonomic function. However, it is scarcely scientific to assume that the autonomic system in isolation could lose its equilibrium, as the term 'autonomic dystonia' suggests.

The doctor's fear of not being equal to his own personal emotional involvement may cause him to resort to polypharmacy. Patients complaining of tiredness are prescribed without further ado vitamins, anabolic agents and 'tonics', although they only have a placebo effect. This was shown by Bugard (quoted in Maeder 1953) in double-blind trials. The doctor frequently prescribes a psychotropic drug in order to calm himself – but it is the patient who must swallow it.

This tendency is now quite rightly contested. It is true that tranquilizers eliminate the inner tension caused by unresolved conflicts and problems. They do not, of course, solve the problems themselves. On the contrary, the drugs deprive a person of the opportunity to evolve through inner tension and rob him of one of the most important conditions and prerequisites for true personality development and maturation. Thus regular consumption of high doses of psychotropic drugs could eventually result in the loss of the distinguishing feature of a normal, healthy person – personal freedom.

A 48-year-old 'exhausted' patient was referred to us from Italy; she had been treated by eighteen doctors over a period of two and a half years. On admission she brought with her 2.4 kg of drugs that had been prescribed for her. Some of the packs had not even been opened and they covered the whole of her bedside table. Before writing a prescription, particularly a repeat prescription, the doctor should bear in mind that behind indeterminate complaints may lurk a desire on the part of the patient to have a personal relationship with his physician.

If the psychosocial condition of the patient is not taken into account and purely objective clinical aspects are allowed to assume total importance to the exclusion of everything else, the patient will be pinned down into a simplifying pattern of 'cause and effect' and relegated to a passive *object of treatment*. He will then supposedly be '*made*' healthy again. The patient's own efforts involving his inherent capacities of self-regulation and self-healing, i.e. his active participation, will beome stunted though neglect. The impression is sometimes gained that such capacities are thought to impede a 'smooth-running' treatment.

Many patients today have the attitude that their illness is a matter for the health insurance and the doctor: it is their business to deal with the expensive affliction, not the patient's. He remains the objective spectator. Yet it is the patient's *subjective attitude* to the illness that is important during its entire course.

M. Bleuler (1969) pointed out that faulty conceptions of illness and ill-conceived terms or expressions can severely affect health: 'We like to think that medical terms are concerned only with facts, forgetting that we often imbue them with overtones and distortion that can do harm. The classic example of this is Charcot's concept of hysteria. This great neurologist and teacher was convinced that hysteria must be distinguished by a characteristic set of symptoms, as he had discovered to be the case with multiple sclerosis. In his eager efforts to delimit a uniform 'hysteria' syndrome, he created such a syndrome. Under his influence the young girls in the Salpêtrière became *grandes hystériques*, became contorted by severe convulsions and hemialgia, and proved astonishingly responsive to hypnosis. In accordance with his concept of hysteria, so developed hysteria before his eyes. A dramatic syndrome came into being – and he could not have wished for a better one to include in his world-famous clinical lectures.'

Even many insurance schemes show a bias in favour of terms expressing physical illness. They tend to reward efforts expended in purely technical spheres but fail to take into account the time taken up by a personal approach. The American family doctor Greco (Greco and Pittenger) reported how his income dropped after employing the psychosomatic approach learned in Balint groups. True, he derived greater satisfaction from his work, but the prospect of a drop in income hardly encourages a doctor to venture into this field, particularly after having gone to the trouble of training himself and having to cope with inital feelings of uncertainty.

10.2 Various Forms of Dialogue with the Patient

Doctors have always attributed great importance to a dialogue with the patient, if only for the purpose of history taking. They know that if insufficient progress is made at this stage it will be necessary to talk to the patient all over again about symptoms and past history.

We have used the word 'dialogue'. But a closer look at the usual structure and character of this interview shows that it cannot always be called a dialogue in the strict sense. What in effect happens is that the patient describes his symptoms and these immediately conjure up a picture in the doctor's mind of the disorder from which he might be suffering. On the basis of this picture the doctor then asks further questions with a view to either reinforcing his first impressions or refuting them. The patient makes an effort to describe his symptoms, his subjective experience. But the doctor proceeds in a specific direction, and it is he who takes the lead. Jung considered this to be a common fault of the insensitive physician.

This is, moreover, not a true dialogue. It is merely a questioning of the patient by the doctor; for the patient is completely unaware of the purpose of the conversation, and the doctor, who has a general picture of possible disorders in his mind, attempts to fit the patient's symptoms into this pattern. Only at a relatively late stage does one make the great discovery that far more can be learnt about things that really motivate the patient if, instead of asking him questions, one lets him describe what is going through his mind, i.e. if one simply listens and does not interrupt. In such an interview the doctor is interested not only in the symptoms but in the patient's life. In the true dialogue quality is more important than quantity.

Condrau describes the following types of doctor-patient dialogue:

1. *The Trivial Interview*. This type of conversation, which occurs all too often during consultations, is meaningless since it makes use of 'killer phrases', truisms which at best serve to obscure other truths ('We're only human', or 'everybody has something wrong with him'). A similar tendency is to identify with the patient ('How are we today?', 'The weather affects me, too') and play down his complaints ('It's not as bad as it seems', 'You can bear it').
2. *The Psychagogic Interview*. Direct questions are put to the doctor. He is asked for advice about marriage or jobs or about bringing up children, and his opinion is sought on problems of social and philosophical interest. This type of conversation gives impetus to the doctor's need to play an active part and is therefore a great source of satisfaction. In certain situations it is eminently suitable; however, it also has its bad points since the nature of any advice is determined by the personality structure of the therapist and therefore does not necessarily fit the needs of the patient, as, for example, when a doctor recommends a sexually inhibited patient with erythrophobia to visit a prostitute or advises an obviously guilt-ridden patient with a masturbation complex to look within himself and repent.
3. *The Authoritarian Interview*. It is not uncommon for a doctor to be held in great esteem and to enjoy great renown since his enterprise and self-assurance can make him a figure of authority. The patient feels secure and protected in the shelter of this authority. Authoritarian interviews are conducted in particular by doctors who prefer not to discuss their instructions. The psychological effect of such instructions rests on their suggestive character and stands or falls with the measure prescribed.

4. *The Understanding Interview*. This can be specific (focal therapy) or open-ended. It is conflict-related, that is to say, related to the patient's worries and problems: his case history and life history are discussed with him, the patient being allowed as far as possible to take the lead in the conversation. A dialogue of this type can be either psychotherapeutic or preparative to psychotherapy. A patient should never be referred to a psychiatrist unless such an understanding, empathetic conversation has taken place.
5. *The 'Enlightening', Analytical Interview*. This should be conducted only by a specialist in psychotherapy. The techniques of this type of interview cannot be learned from books or courses. It is an open-ended conversation which in addition to free association includes the interpretation of dreams and fantasies. Conversations of this type usually extend over a period of months or years and are indicated particularly in severe neurotic character disturbances but also in chronic psychosomatic disorders.

Every meeting with the doctor has its effect on the patient. He feels the difference between a dialogue in which his personality, hopes, expectations and disappointments are of significance and one in which he is merely asked to give as full an account as possible of past illnesses and accidents. If the patient detects this *communicative resonance* on the part of the doctor, the treatment can be enhanced to a surprising degree. The revelatory power inherent in such a dialogue helps the patient far more than quick explanations and advice – even when such information is 'correct'.

10.3 Function and Course of the Interview

Whatever its origin, a somatic disturbance will always constitute a reservoir of emotional tension. Every practitioner is aware of the importance of learning to assess the patient's emotional stability before embarking on any specific treatment.

'The doctor should approach the patient with neither presumption nor commotion', wrote the German general practitioner Matthias Wehring in 1818. Very few patients will pour out their hearts at the first opportunity, yet generally they are just waiting for someone to give them a signal to talk about their real problems – even those of a very intimate nature; they are eager for the sense of relief this will bring them. After such an encounter they are better able to bear the human distress expressed in their symptoms.

One may not dismiss a patient lightly by saying that he is not really ill, that there is 'nothing really wrong' with him or that it is 'just nerves'. We must be fair to our patients; they deserve to have their complaints taken seriously, without prejudice or reservation, even when no physical cause can be discovered. The symptom should be respected during the diagnostic phase; after all, it is not only experienced on an organic plane, but – and this is the point – on an emotional one too. It often serves as a form of relief to patients under great tension.

Therapy embodying a specific aim must be carried out in a spirit of partnership, equal value being accorded to the work on hand and to the relationship. Surgeons say: we must make the patient an ally in our therapy. It will be readily understood that any drugs prescribed after a discussion have a different kind of effect than after a summary consultation. The first consultation where there is opportunity for conversation need not last any longer than usual. It may constitute the beginning of therapy and therefore be of extreme significance to both doctor and patient.

'Opening Moves'

Many authors have stressed the importance of putting the patient at ease, i.e. giving him time to adjust to the atmosphere of the first interview. Balint (1968) has likened this to the opening moves in chess. They constitute a neutral prelude to the conversation, consisting, for example, of a few impersonal questions about the patient's journey or a short chat about the weather. Such a neutral start also means that the patient's first impression of us is gained in a calm, informal atmosphere. Questions about who referred the patient to us or how he came to hear of us can also easily be incorporated in the opening moves. All this need only take a few minutes.

The second stage of the interview involves direct questions about the reason for the patient's visit. Langen suggests the doctor should say, for example: 'What seems to be the trouble?' or 'What brings you here?'. The form of the question should be adapted to the type of person involved and his background. A conscious effort should be made to avoid mentioning pain, complaints or illness in these nonspecific questions. It is particularly important to avoid suggestive questions. Questioning should be directed towards the person as a whole.

The doctor must take note of both verbal and averbal modes of expression on the part of the patient; this means not only listening but keeping one's eyes open too. The following facts and details can prove informative from the very beginning: the patient's manner when the consultation is being arranged; whether he is late or early for his appointment; critical or passive behaviour while waiting; extreme communicativeness with the staff; his opening remarks; his style of dress; whether he comes alone or needs the protection of friends or members of his family; hair style, facial expression, gestures, handshake; where and how the patient sits down; his tone of voice and choice of words; whether he is talkative, continually sighing, silent, provocative, hostile, rebellious or approachable.

The initiative should ideally come from the patient. During gaps in the conversation, described by Moser as *affective nodal points*, the patient is examining the doctor. Is the doctor a person who will listen and who can be trusted to keep a secret? The doctor may be thinking: 'This is a boring story - I've heard it all before', or 'difficult case, this'. The patient watches his face to see whether it expresses severity or warmth. A reciprocal analysis of the situation takes place even before the actual conversation begins.

The people who visit us are usually restless and tense because they have to talk about something they have rarely, if ever, discussed before. They may see the doctor as some sort of 'body technician', or even as a sage or magician. In any case, they expect something of his abilities or wisdom.

The patients usually relax during the first minutes. They are almost amazed how easy it is to talk about normal problems and are surprised to find they can discuss even those of the most personal nature without feeling uncomfortable or embarrassed.

It is particularly useful if the doctor can introduce an unexpected turn in the conversation which will perplex most patients. Meerwein (1960) writes: 'When the patient has described his physical complaints the doctor asks his opinion on the cause. The question comes as a surprise and, like any other surprise, will release emotions which would otherwise have remained hidden. For the patient will usually assume that the doctor regards himself as the only person competent to answer this question and will be all the more prepared to leave this task to him since it will guarantee the continuing concealment of the conflict by the symptom.'

The More Concentrated Interview

The *first interview* is very important in determining the subsequent course of the doctor-patient relationship. One's own emotional reactions should be used right from the outset as a diagnostic and therapeutic aid. Sometimes the patient will try to solve his problems himself by employing his habitual system of transference and defence.

The patient should be regarded as a 'subject' and not as an 'object'. The greater the emotional component in the patient's illness, the greater in general will be the doctor's own emotional involvement; he may feel particularly sympathetic towards the patient or be annoyed by him and find him disagreeable. He must, however, recognize this as a personal reaction and keep it under control by means of increased self-awareness. He must always be aware of what is happening between himself and the patient. He must be 'daring' in thought, have 'mad' ideas and yet be circumspect in his actions.

According to Kind, 'the busy doctor is particularly prone to giving advice too hastily and at too early a stage in the conversation, thus acting on the basis of incomplete or preconceived knowledge of the patient. A responsible attitude is first to listen and to let the patient speak so that he can formulate his problem – as much for his own benefit as for the doctor's. Very often the patient becomes aware of his worries and conflicts only when he has to explain the reason for his visit.'

From the outset the conversation must also have a therapeutic aim; the patient must be able to sense this, for he often wants to be treated from the moment he enters the consulting room.

The doctor who knows how to listen not only enables his patient to elaborate on his symptoms but also allows him to give expression to his attitude to the world, his preferences, his hidden aggressions and his secret desires.

The patient must feel that he can talk without fear of being judged or condemned. He should feel that he can tend to be somewhat aggressive without erecting a barrier between himself and the doctor. For he does want to confide. He may perhaps come to know his deepest feelings for the first time when he realizes that the doctor is interested in him and when he senses the doctor's aim to integrate the symptom into his own life.

It should be left to the patient to take the initiative in the conversation; this can be done, for example, by using Deutsch's 'associative anamnesis' technique (1939, 1964), which allows the patient to oscillate continuously between the mental and the physical poles. At first the patient gives information only about his organic disturbances, after which he usually holds back and expects to be asked questions. One must take care not to miss the right moment at which to introduce a key word into the discussion. At this point the doctor will repeat one of the last things said by the patient in the form of a question. The patient will then usually give further details of his complaints and also speak of things that give information about his emotional life as well as his organic condition. Thus he himself will often relate his somatic symptoms to his emotional life, his environment and his relationsips with other people.

Extreme importance attaches to the way in which a question is formulated by the doctor. A less specific question offers greater scope for association and is therefore to be preferred. A question that is too precise, however, restricts the answers that are possible and jeopardizes the spontaneity of the conversation. It may nevertheless help the patient along when he comes to a problem that he lacks the courage to tackle; thus in some circumstances we may arrive at an answer obliquely, and this always yields interesting information about the patient's unconscious associations.

However important it may be what the doctor says, it is even more important how he says it. What is absolutely decisive, however, is when he says it. According to Wiesenhütter, the present-day psychotherapist is becoming 'largely an advocate and practitioner of silence'. Our everyday expressions are indicative of the various types of silence that are possible: in a positive sense silence can be astonished, attentive, spellbound or awestruck, and in a negative sense heavy, embarrassed, awkward, painful, wounding, icy or deathly. Bewilderment, surprise, embarrassment, helplessness, and even ineffable friendship can all find expression in silence. Any hasty attempt on the part of the doctor to get the patient to talk usually has the opposite effect and merely serves to reinforce his defensive attitude. Just as words can be meaningless, so can silence be full of meaning. And just as language involves speaking, listening and being silent, so it can be said that the conversation between doctor and patient consists in talking to each other, listening to each other and at times in being in silent communion.

10.4 The Dialogue as an Aid to Therapy

Does the doctor in private practice really have enough time to conduct the more intense form of interview? 'How can one make time when apparently there isn't any?' asks Meier, and then goes on to say: 'As you can imagine, it is impossible to carry on a relaxed conversation with the patient if there are twenty people in the waiting room next door talking and coughing expectantly. Our working day must be arranged in such a way that set amounts of time are alloted to house calls, routine consultations and talking to patients with psychic complaints. Each of the latter requires up to an hour to relax, thaw out and realize that the doctor not only recognizes their problems but is also understanding towards them.'

Patients frequently suffer from psychosocial conflicts that cannot be solved by the doctor but only by themselves. The doctor can nevertheless be of great help in his role of understanding partner. During the course of client-centred therapy one continually observes that, even without giving direct advice or appealing to rational understanding, the problems and conflicts lose their intensity – often because the patient is merely ready to accept them.

The conversation that takes place in the doctor's surgery is not a simple form of dialogue, nor is it simple medicine. It is precisely in this type of approach to the patient that we make a particularly personal commitment.

Schlegel writes: 'Mentally one must take off one's white coat. I made it my practice to put down my pen, push the patient's file to one side, cross my legs and fold my arms. The result of these experiments was that cases became acquaintances. What was "just one more case" became an individual; a member of the human species became a fellowman. Or, referring to the situation, a consultation became a meeting. I now knew something of the fate of my patients, of their character and of the way in which they reacted to their destiny. From then on they were more than just cases, since fate and character mark everyone as a unique individual. Perhaps it could be said that I was sympathetic towards these patients. But then "sympathy" is not synonymous with compassion, as is often superficially assumed – "sympathy" means "feeling-with". In many respects their fate and character were similar to my own, in other respects the opposite. I recognized my fellowmen as the product of other human destinies. It is as though I had said to myself: "Given the same parents and exposed to the same fate, I would now be like this patient."

'A case became an acquaintance – but what is an acquaintance, a friend? We doctors should know – for most of us distinguish clearly between whether we are treating patients or treating relatives and friends.'

It is particularly important that the doctor should not have any illusions when setting the aims of treatment. Excessive optimism and confidence can become the root of frustration, and this in turn can cause tension, for both the doctor and the patient, which may destroy the relationship that has been built up between them.

The aims of treatment can range from symptomatic management and affective support to complete restoration of the psychophysical equilibrium. However, in the majority of cases, particularly in those involving neurotic maladjustment, it is wiser to settle for a result some way between these two extremes: one hopes for something more than an abatement of the symptoms but does not expect complete recovery.

Many questions remain open. For example: How can this rapprochement between doctor and patient prevent the fixation of symptoms? When does it become the actual gateway to psychotherapy? And what types of psychotherapy should subsequently be employed?

For the doctor intending to use short-term psychotherapy it may be useful to know the main prerequisites for this method of treatment: In addition to his general training and the necessary specialized knowledge the doctor must possess the ability to understand the 'whisperings of the unconscious' and also have the necessary mental agility to practice different therapeutic techniques at the same time. Added to this are his personal quality, inner readiness and real desire to help, and his full acknowledgement of the restricted resources and the needs of the patient.

We conclude this section with an extract from Bleuler's essay (1970) *Bleiben wir am Kranken* (Let's keep to the patient): 'It is sad to think that we could relieve the anxieties and worries of many patients if we had more time for them. We should then need fewer pain-killers, sleeping pills and tranquilizers, and probably fewer purgatives and tonics; we might even be able to give diabetics less insulin or to spare a pregnant women a perineal tear. If we consoled and relaxed our patients we could do a great deal for them. We could promote sleep or stimulate appetite and digestion. We also know that for at least a quarter of our patients, performing a physical examination serves only as a means of excluding physical therapeutic indications and that the only help that can be given to these patients, if any, is psychotherapeutic. The depressing question is, how many of those whom we could help with psychotherapy do we really help?

'Nowadays we are well aware how much personal medical care means to the patient – we talk and write about it all the time.

'The doctor-patient relationship in the foreground of the therapeutic process has basic therapeutic significance in itself, added to which suggestive and psychocathartic forces are at work within it. It facilitates counseling. It creates good conditions for relaxation, clarification, self-discovery and maturation of the personality. For this reason alone we would not be completely unjustified in classing what radiates from the doctor's personality to the patient during physical treatment under the heading of psychotherapy.

'What should the individual doctor do to prevent isolation of the patient? What is his psychotherapy in the broad sense of the word? First and foremost he must want to be with his patient. He must spend a little more time with him, talk to him a little more and on occasions introduce into the conversation a warmer and more personal note than a physical disorder would call for. This alone will afford the patient some relief. By mitigating despair and emotional excitation, the doctor can often also reduce autonomic excitation and tension and improve muscle tone, respiration, blood pressure, sleep. If he approaches the patient on a personal level he will win him over to his physical diagnosis and therapy and at the same time find ways and means of ensuring that his advice is followed. He will then be in a position to find the right words and right tone to use with any patient whether he is educated or uneducated, intelligent or unintelligent, anxious or calm. He will not recommend to a member of a family a diet that the housewife cannot prepare; he will not recommend costly treatment to a patient who cannot afford it; he will be more likely to advise that a sick child should be admitted to hospital if he knows that the mother does not look after it properly and *vice versa*; he will be more likely to find the correct approach to a patient's partner if he is aware of the state of their marital relationship; when issuing a medical certificate for the employer, he will be better able to do justice to the patient's disorder and his needs if he has some knowledge of the atmosphere at work and his relationship with his employer. These things, and many others like them, however, are only possible if the doctor has come to know the patient as a person and is not simply interested in his disorder. If the patient feels that the doctor is taking his personal circumstances into consideration, then the association between the two of them will become even closer and gain in therapeutic value.'

10.5 Balint Groups

Does the doctor in private practice really have enough time to have a more intensive dialogue with his patients? Does he in fact possess sufficient skill? Potentially, yes. There appears to exist a form of prescientific understanding of psychosomatic correlations in the art of medicine. It is part and parcel of the stock of knowledge of every self-respecting family doctor who 'knows his customers'. 'Common-sense psychology' has always been employed by doctors when, for example, they have had occasion to advise patients to take a rest, change their occupation, pull themselves together or leave home.

M. Balint (1957) emphasized that such recommendations were often by no means wrong but thought it a mistake to conclude that an experienced physician had enough knowledge of everyday psychology to deal effectively with his patients' emotional conflicts and personality problems. No surgeon would under normal circumstances perform minor surgery with, say, a kitchen knife or a woodworking tool, no matter how efficient such implements were in their right place.

The doctor really needs guidance and occasional check-ups on results, which frequently show that he knows much more than thinks. Such knowledge can be called upon, being, as it were, preconscious (Knoepfel).

M. Balint accordingly developed a system of training, primarily for doctors, in groups. This was based on the realization that the doctor's own personality, feelings and reactions constitute an important diagnostic and therapeutic instrument. Balint groups are concerned with the use of this aid and the difficult matter of administering the correct 'dosage' of what has been called the 'drug doctor'.

A Balint group consists of ten to twelve physicians and a group leader. In recent years Balint groups have also been set up for non-doctors, particularly for nursing staff, social workers, physiotherapists, clinical psychologists and even for theologists and members of other professions. The group leader is usually a psychotherapist and occasionally a very experienced physician with the right background. The main requirement for doctors attending the course is that they exercise their profession and have continual and direct contact to patients. The sessions are held weekly or twice monthly over a period of several years. The duration of an individual session is two hours. Each group should retain as far as possible the same participants. There is usually an emotionally free atmosphere of friendly solidarity in which one may even risk making a fool of oneself with impunity.

Balint groups differ from a normal training course in that the experience of the participants is given prominence. They are thus not self-awareness groups in the usual sense since the self-awareness is closely bound up with and related to dealing with patients.

The ability to be acquired largely comprises that necessary for developing and understanding a doctor-patient relationship. At the same time family constellations and psychosocial problems are taken into account (Petzold 1984a,b, 1988a). The participants take turns in relating cases encountered in daily practice. These should be as recent as possible since the emotional participation of the doctor is then at its strongest. Balint once suggested selecting the third case of the previous day as a rule of thumb in order to avoid the tendency of seeking out problem patients only. When details of the case have been given, it is discussed by the group.

The doctor must discover his own ability to spy out certain things concerning his patients that are hardly possible to express in words, and must consequently begin by 'eavesdropping' on the same sort of language within himself (Balint 1955). He will relive the case while describing it and will already become consciously aware of many of his feelings and reactions relating to the patient, even though these had escaped him at the time.

It frequently becomes apparent that every doctor has a vague but fairly set idea of how a person behaves when sick. Although this idea is far from concrete, it is incredibly stubborn and permeates practically all aspects of the doctor's work with his patients (Balint 1957a). Preferences, ambitions, unconscious sympathy or antipathy, prejudices and psychic defence mechanisms all come to light.

In order to get on better with his patients the doctor must become aware of his own set patterns of behaviour influencing the doctor–patient relationship and gradually obtain at least some measure of independence from them. This makes him more open and accessible to the patient. At the same time he is able to achieve a degree of distance from the patient and offer the empathy required by a sick person in order to open up and cooperate.

With increasing knowledge of his own personality the doctor becomes aware of his own influence as a 'drug', including both the therapeutic and side effects. He learns how to exert this influence at a more conscious level, how to administer the correct dosage and choose his words on an individual basis. Moreover, he will no longer be so easy to manipulate by patients who want him all for themselves. He will also be prepared to take the risk of his patients discharging their emotional feelings to obtain relief from tension and be able to cope better with aggressivity.

It is not the practice in Balint groups to bore into the ultimate depths of the doctors participating; pride of place is given to analysing observations made in routine practice that the doctor continually records but which do not mean much to him. Reliving experiences while describing a case can be of help in recalling details overlooked during consultations and treatment. The group leader and other participants point out items of information supplied by the patient that failed to find any echo on the part of the doctor, or peculiarities of speech, facial expressions and gestures that either go unnoticed or are misinterpreted by those untrained in this field.

Discussing a case with the group will also make the doctor increasingly aware of certain behavioural patterns on the part of the patient that disturb the doctor–patient relationship. He learns to recognize the patient's resistance for what it is and to take heed of the social situation prevailing at the time of the illness, particularly of factors relating to the family and work. It is then frequently found that a conflict situation exists. The discussions make it easier for the doctor to get a better picture of the role played by the symptoms 'proposed' and sense what the patient expects of him. In other words, he must also be able to interpret the patient's complaint.

An important experience made in group discussions is how a certain basic mood or ambivalent attitude of the patient is brought to light.

Widely differing opinions on the patient usually point to a high degree of ambivalence on his part. Long years of practice in this field teach the doctor to make use of his various reactions to the patient. Such reactions help him grasp the essentials of the patient's personality structure and can be employed as a diagnostic aid.

Even discussions on the different ways of handling patients and hearing how other participants do this can open up new aspects of behaviour to individual doctors.

Balint attributed great importance to the group leader. If he finds the right manner and tone of leading his particular group, his didactic value will be greater than that of all the other participants together. After all, the techniques advocated are based on a special type of listening that doctors are supposed to acquire from him. If the group leader allows each participant to be himself, to speak how and when he wants, and to gain the impression that he himself has found *one* correct way of handling the patient's problems (and not been prescribed *the* correct way), it will then be possible to illustrate in the 'here and now' situation what there is to learn (Balint 1955).

The objection is often made that Balint groups take up too much of the busy practitioner's time. Although it is true that attendance at the sessions incurs sacrificing some time, in the long run time can actually be saved. A doctor with this training behind him is able to perceive far quicker why a patient consults him, and avoid much waste of time in beating about the bush. There is far less 'confusion of tongues', namely the clash of different automatic patterns of behaviour on the part of doctor and patient.

Balint (1957a,b, 1968) illustrated this by taking the diagnosis as an example. He distinguished between three levels of diagnosis:

1. The traditional diagnosis based on study of the disease (e.g. essential hypertension, rheumatoid arthritis).
2. Consideration of why the patient has chosen this particular time to visit us or to request a house call, of the real reasons behind this 'offer' to the doctor.
3. Finally, the 'overall diagnosis' which, in addition to the disorder, is centred on the whole patient and embraces his psychological, social and character-related conflicts.

The traditional diagnosis typifies modern medical science, the prime aim of which is to work out diagnostic and therapeutic methods by which organic disease can be recognized and treated.

People with illnesses that can be diagnosed and treated by medical, scientific techniques only are included by Balint (1965) under 'class I diseases'. He distinguishes these patients from those 'who are themselves ill' and allocates their complaints to 'class II diseases'. There are of course 'mixed cases'.

The clinical picture of a disease is everything that the doctor is able to observe in his patient. Yet only what the doctor considers important enough to warrant as part of the illness will be relevant for treatment.

An appraisal thus takes place that may be blurred or distorted by the items that can be observed and those actually observed. Both observation and appraisal are largely determined by the manner in which a doctor has been trained, i.e. 'what medicine is for him'.

Given certain conditions of training this may mean that 'class II diseases' cannot be diagnosed or that the diagnosis made does not coincide with the patient's actual state.

A sequel to a wrong diagnosis is a form of interplay between doctor and patient. This may consist of examinations, drug therapy and dietary prescriptions on the part of the doctor, and the most varying symptoms on that of the patient. According to Balint this interplay may continue till doctor and patient enter into a tacit collusion. For 'class I diseases' this 'compromise' means that a diagnosis has been made and an appropriate therapy found. Should doctor and patient reach an agreement that a 'class II disease' is a 'class I disease' the result will be a pseudo-diagnosis and the treatment a mere placebo. Balint considered that since no true diagnosis is possible in such circumstances the 'compromise' is really being treated and not the illness.

Such a development can be avoided only when the doctor is able to make an overall diagnosis, i.e. that his attention is directed not only to the complaint with which the patient presents but to the 'whole man'.

Experience has borne out that this is no mere theoretical consideration. Reports such as the following are by no means rare:

> 'Over a period of several years – and after attempts at diagnosis by an internist, a specialist in respiratory disease, a gynecologist and a surgeon who had recommended an appendectomy – the patient came to consult me practically every week with the most varying complaints. Sometimes it was pain in the right intestinal cavity, sometimes in the back. She almost drove me crazy with her seemingly trivial talk, which went on and on even when I had my hands full. The stubborn back pain occasioned me to refer her to a well-known orthopedist. He reported that the range of movement was normal, although there was a slight tenderness in the muscles of the lumbar region, and prescribed a course of physiotherapy.
>
> 'But she continued to come to see me regularly during my hours of consultation once a week, and, to my consternation, began to flirt with me rather aggressively. One day I told her abruptly that there was nothing very much that I do for her any longer and thought it would be better if she resumed her work as a sales assistant and did not appear again in my surgery for a certain time. It was two years before I saw here again. She came to me with the same complaints with a sort of

childish remorse. ("Did you miss me? I hope you're not still annoyed with me.") Then she appeared every week as before and recommenced flirting with me, sought contact with my foot under the desk and placed her hand on mine. I corrected her and she wept. But she continued to appear weekly, received five to ten minutes conversation and a bottle of medicine.

'Thanks to my increasing understanding of personality disturbances she finally received a full hour's consultation, during which, among many other things, she told me about her childhood; about her father in the navy who was rarely home; of her affection for a younger brother who died about the time her symptoms appeared; of her dyspareunia from the very beginning of her marriage, and of her complete incapacity for sexual intercourse since her brother's death. Further investigations are under way. Since this longer conversation her attitude towards me has changed considerably. She no longer attempts to flirt with me and there has been some improvement in her symptoms. But four years and an appendectomy were needed before I found time for that hour's consultation. *Mea culpa!*' (Balint 1955).

Many patients ask their doctor to make a house call – often at night – if he fails to assess correctly the symptoms they 'propose'. There is an old German proverb that says: 'He that will not hear must be made to feel.' We could change this slightly to fit the case and say: 'He that cannot hear must jump to it!' Generally speaking, the doctor who has attended Balint groups not only saves time but has a less hectic practice.

Greco, the American doctor mentioned on p. 179 who received a thorough training in a Balint group, similarly reported a time-saving in daily routine practice. He acquired the ability of listening to his patients and achieved more productive results during his hours of consultation even though he spent more time on *individual* patients. His income dropped initially by a third because the number of patients visiting him at the surgery was reduced by half. 'There is more time. I don't make quite so much money. It's worth it.' Greco sees his personal gain, however, in the fact that he can now deal with his 'problem patients' in a manner similar to that in which he treats those with organic disorders. Emotional disorders are no longer such a worry to him. He has the feeling of having achieved something that corresponds closer to earlier ideas and conceptions that prompted him to become a practitioner. His deeper understanding of the patients and their families has increased the satisfaction he derives from his daily practice and he feels he has gained in personal maturity.

The advantages of acquiring this solid basis in minor psychotherapy may be summarized at this juncture. It enables the general practitioner to achieve the following:

- To recognize and straighten out a problematic doctor-patient relationship charged with conflicts (Luban-Plozza and Loch).

- To diagnose unresolved psychogenic, psychosomatic and psychosocial conflicts in his patients before it is too late and understand the dynamics of an individual case of illness in this context.
- To administer treatment individually and always within a different framework of reference (Stucke) – and to keep a firm hold on his own attitude and problems.

Junior Balint groups (Luban-Plozza 1974; Luban-Plozza and Balint 1978) for medical students have now been in existence at various universities since 1969, the first experiences being made in Milan. These groups consist of fifth and sixth year students, who have already had personal experience of attending to patients during practical training and night duty (in some countries they volunteer for such work either out of financial reasons or to supplement their rather theoretically biased studies with practical experience). We therefore experienced no particular difficulty during the sessions in finding a volunteer to report on the case under discussion. The aim of these groups is to impart an understanding of the patient's illness and contributing factors by common efforts to make an overall diagnosis. This helps students establish the all important interpersonal relationship with patients (Kröger and Luban-Plozza). The group leader has an additional role here of overcoming any problems peculiar to the student situation by exercising a more didactic function. Schüffel (1978) and Bregulla-Beyer are of the opinion that 'history-taking groups' can supplement this form of training.

Balint groups modelled on the annual international meetings held in Ascona, Switzerland, promote contact between students, hospital doctors, general practitioners, and university lecturers. The encounter of people in different phases of life and development provides all participants with a host of new ideas and experience. This is extended and increased in depth by the partial inclusion of patients, who have the opportunity of expressing a personal view of their illness and its history (Luban-Plozza 1989).

11 The Rudiments of Treatment

11.1 The Problems of Integrating Psychotherapeutic Principles Into General Medicine

In his daily contact with patients the general practitioner constantly finds himself face to face with this dilemma: On the one hand, he has learnt to see his task in interpreting objective findings, for which a broad palette of scientific methodology and apparatus are at his disposal; on the other, he is all too often bound to admit that this kind of diagnostic procedure provides no satisfactory answer to the patient's complaint.

The primary cause of this situation lies in the way medicine has developed and that psychology failed to do so along parallel lines. While medicine evolved into an experimental science, psychology, by recognizing the significance of suggestion and adhering to its own laws, retained its magical associations much longer. This explains the resistance to the introduction of psychology into medicine, and also accounts for the hitherto second-class status of psychology in medical training. It must have seemed like a foreign body and a hindrance to scientific progress. Given the earlier concept of medicine as a natural science, medical courses were necessarily hostile to psychology.

This attitude is still not completely outmoded. True, it is now generally accepted that the patient must be regarded as a somatopsychic whole and that a truly patient-orientated medicine should take into account the relationships between physical and emotional processes; but what in fact remains is training provided in the various specialties, among which persists the second-class status of psychological aspects.

There is generally little opportunity for establishing personal relationships with patients during the period of study. The student is presented with the illness as being the object of medicine. Yet it is the patient who has the illness, and patients are subjects. These doctors in the making are later confronted with the difficulty of creating an association between subject and object. From that moment on, they are largely 'on their own'.

It is precisely this form of initiation that makes it difficult for psychotherapeutic methods to gain a foothold in professional medical practice. This is based on a hierarchical system which relies on the division of labour among specialists in order to gather the elements for a final synthesis. Such a system undoubtedly has its advantages; each examination is the responsibility of scientifically qualified specialists and both time and money can be saved. It results, however, in a fragmented picture of medicine, with the patient being regarded as nothing more than a collection of organs and systems. Furthermore, the doctor-patient relationship often becomes impersonal and formal since the patient has little opportunity to build up a close relationship with a particular doctor and thus lacks real human contact.

The increasing need for a medical approach that is directed towards the whole man does not spring from theoretical deliberations but from shortcomings constantly encountered in general practice by doctors and patients alike.

Doctors are becoming increasingly aware that their efforts to help their patients lead them not only into the more familiar somatic field but also into the less well-known territory of psychosocial reactions. This task can be mastered only by employing a *multifactorial approach*, a sociopsychosomatic approach in fact, since this alone is capable of pinpointing the pathogenic cause of disorders of this type amid the 'dynamic interference' which is always to be found between organic, subjective and social forces.

The young doctor, particularly the young general practitioner, is usually inadequately prepared for such a task. Even with increasing experience, the necessary know-how does not come of its own accord. Cooper cited three major difficulties encountered by general practitioners faced with their patients' psychic problems: lack of time, a pessimistic attitude towards problems of this type, and a false impression of their own role in relation to psychiatry.

11.2 Relationship Therapy

The general practitioner can usually exert a greater psychotherapeutic effect than he realizes, but his knowledge of it is generally prescient and unsystematic. His full capacity in this field thus remains undeveloped. At the same time the general practitioner has excellent chances of getting to know the patient's psychosocial situation and apply his influence by dint of his close contacts with many patients and their families. In our opinion he should by all means take full advantage of these chances. As we have repeatedly pointed out, however, 'common sense' by itself is not enough. The practitioner needs to acquire the knowledge and skill of applying the necessary techniques and to develop a 'therapeutic personality'.

Psychological knowledge is essential in order to make a correct assessment of the patient's psychodynamic peculiarities and to understand what the symptoms are trying to express. The doctor must also be able to form a clear picture of the reciprocal influences exerted by himself and his patient.

Every interpersonal relationship and every individual's attitude depends on the *emotional state of those involved.* It is therefore imperative for the doctor to be aware of his own emotions and their basic mechanisms. Only in this way is it possible to ensure that there are no signs of personal immaturity to exert a negative effect on his contact with the patient.

The patient's unconscious expectations of the doctor and the doctor's reactions to them are particularly significant. Both are accorded great importance in relationship therapy.

Psychological training for the general practitioner should be centred around the diagnostic possibilities presented by the relationship in the sense of interaction and cooperation. The aim is to enable the general practitioner to recognize and interpret the sort of relationship existing and the patient's social network; these factors can then be taken into account in the diagnosis and be incorporated into the process we have called *relationship therapy.* A doctor's reactions towards the patient can provide valuable clues as to the latter's condition if the doctor is aware of such reactions and able to interpret them.

The case-to-case self-awareness acquired in Balint groups or under individual supervision in postgraduate psychotherapy courses is essential for doctors employing psychosomatic principles. It constitutes, moreover, a firm basis for understanding the theoretical concepts of the psychodynamic processes involved.

The Doctor's Behaviour

The problems of a psychological nature arising in daily practice are multifarious. Even the initial contact with the patient comprising history taking requires acute powers of observation and a good deal of circumspection on the part of the doctor. This has to be combined with the ability to build up a strong bond of trust so that the patient feels free to voice his needs without reserve. Unintentional omissions or untrue statements are sometimes to be explained by motives of a depth psychological character, which the doctor should be in a position to recognize (Luban-Plozza et al. 1987).

Everything the doctor says is important in gaining the patient's trust, regardless of whether he is discussing details of the illness itself, a possible operation, diet or drug therapy. The way in which a drug is described to the patient is at least as important as what is actually written on the prescription. When our *angina temporis*, precipitated by the sight of an overflowing waiting room, threatens to become acute we should remind ourselves that the words we address to the patient or to his relatives are loaded with dynamite.

Doctors find the passive behaviour required particularly difficult since this does not fit in with their accustomed activity of history taking and performing clinical examinations in the somatic field. Here, taking a case history involves letting the patient talk about what he subjectively considers to be important. A few questions about the course of the disorder and its connections with the patient's life may be of value at a latter stage in the conversation.

The aspects of behaviour dealt with up to this point make it clear that the relationships and mutual reactions between doctor and patient are influenced to a great extent by our behaviour. This constitutes a linchpin for relationship therapy and diagnosis. No amount of experience, no matter how profound, should lull the doctor into a false sense of security; he should never allow his thirst for new facts to be quenched. The doctor-patient relationship must have a firm basis.

Should the nonspecialist find himself in difficulties when faced with vague psychic symptoms or any other unusual situation concerning the diagnosis or treatment arise, he should not hesitate to refer the patient to a psychiatrist. However, it is important to prepare the patient for a consultation of this type so that his meeting with the psychiatrist will occasion as little anxiety as possible. The specialist should then outline in everyday language his suggestions for therapy and where possible lend support to the work of the general practitioner.

The Patient's Behaviour

There are naturally many varied aspects of the patient's behaviour that must be considered. This constitutes the second linchpin in relationship therapy and diagnosis. As a general rule he will try to provoke in the doctor the reaction that suits him. There is often a need for dependence, a typical consequence of the psychic regression which accompanies every illness. This need for dependence is in some patients overt and expressed in their daily life, while others project it onto those with whom they come into contact. Occasionally, this need is expressed in an exaggerated form of aggressivity.

The doctor will not infrequently experience inauspicious, negative or even hostile reactions on the part of the patient. Only if he is aware of the nature of these reactions will the doctor be able to respond to the patient with the understanding and tolerance the situation demands. Lack of trust on the part of the patient is often due to his defensive attitude, which in turn has arisen from an overzealous approach by the doctor, irregular treatment, or disappointment in the doctor. The latter may be unintentional or really desired and dominate the entire relationship. If the doctor understands such defensive attitudes he will be able to keep the patient under control and, if necessary, employ psychotherapeutic 'maintenance therapy'.

A spirit of cooperation on the part of the patient is essential. This cannot, however, simply be demanded on the strength of one's own position and obtained immediately; it is something the doctor must fight for with each successive conversation, and everything depends on the trust he is able to build up between himself and the patient.

Multiple Constellations

We have so far discussed situations involving two persons. But there is an increasing tendency for several people to seek the doctor's attention in a related matter, some directly, others indirectly (Argelander 1963/64, 1966; Ritschl and Luban-Plozza 1987).

This spells added difficulties and constitutes a particular challenge for the general practitioner who also, gets to know the family in every possible situation, can form a picture of them as a whole and discover where their mental and physical strengths and weaknesses lie. His personality has enormous potentialities within all the families he has to meet.

When psychosomatic disturbances are present, the most important questions are: How does the illness of the individual affect the overall family picture? Should the family be treated as a single patient? The doctor is accustomed to concentrate on the individual patient. He tends to overlook that this patient may only be the embodiment of the 'presenting symptom' of a behaviour disturbance within the family as a whole.

Battegay has shown that the psychosomatic disorder of the patient who visits the doctor is often not merely a symptom of the individual but a pathological phenomenon of the whole *group* to which he belongs. The one who acknowledges his condition to the doctor is often simply the one who is conscious of it. In the background there are frequently other members of the family who are ill – the marital partner, siblings, children, parents – or a sick family group whose members are often not consciously aware that they are ill, reject the fact and project it onto those near to them.

A family or equivalent group with a person suffering from a psychosomatic disorder often has a structure based on the sick person's illness. A pathological family equilibrium or norm is established at the expense of the patient, showing a tendency – often a growing tendency – to depart from the norm of the society. Hence, for psychotherapy of psychosomatic patients, the individual cannot be considered in isolation from the group in which he lives. The patient's environment must be taken into account in the doctor's plan of treatment.

Moreover, one must bear in mind the possibility that the symptoms eliminated in a psychosomatic patient can reappear in another member of his family. An explanation for this phenomenon may be that the patient with his complaint often constitutes the mainstay of the unhealthy equilibrium within the family. Every change in the state of the patient's health has been repeatedly shown to have its effect on the collective balance of the group, the members of which are then obliged to find fresh forms of adaptation in order to regain some form of stability.

Even the nonspecialized doctor can exert his positive effect on the family within the concept we have discussed of *family confrontation*. He can, for example, mobilize other members of the family to aid one that has marked emotional disturbances, or help reduce conflictual material that constitutes a strain on the family. The doctor must, however, refrain from laying down the law on how the family should run its life, and neither coax nor conceal. He must learn to wait patiently until the patient or other members of the family can talk, weep or become angry. Patients should be helped to discover *their own* feelings.

Enid Balint devised five groups of questions helpful in clarifying the questions involved, particularly in patients with *marital problems*:

1. How does the patient see himself? How does he see the influence of the key figures in his life (father, mother, siblings, teacher, superiors)?
2. How does the patient see his problems? At the same time, how does the therapist see them?
3. Why did these two people get married? This question is directed at the conscious and unconscious benefits that both partners originally expected to gain. If it cannot be answered, Balint prefers individual psychotherapy.
4. What went wrong in this marriage? Were the hopes on which it was founded fulfilled? What disappointments replaced them?
5. What led the patient to seek help? The story behind the present crisis is usually a long one; why does the patient seek help at this particular time?

Should family confrontation confirm the patient's symptoms to be closely associated with conflict at home and no relief is afforded by the doctor's supportive therapy and counselling, referral is indicated to specialists in family or marriage therapy.

11.3 Methods of Treatment

In determining the treatment indicated for psychosomatic patients one should employ a *pluralistic approach directed towards the patient*. Of the numerous forms of therapy possible, only those should be used that are compatible with the patient's personality structure and his particular illness. The ability of the therapist to carry out the treatment under consideration must also be taken into account, as well as his strongpoints in other methods. It would appear that success in psychotherapy is less a matter of which particular technique is employed so much as whether or not the therapist can deal with the problems that arise.

The following sections should give an overall picture of some of the psychotherapeutic methods applicable to psychosomatic patients.

The Interview (Meerwein 1969)

This lies well within the domain of the family doctor. The know-how and experience needed can be acquired and perfected in Balint groups. In order to help the patient more is needed than a friendly manner and the best of intentions. Only a good knowledge of the typical problems that may arise during illness, together with an understanding for a personal approach to the individual patient, make specific and effective help at all possible.

Experience shows that every conversation with emotionally troubled and tense patients has a cathartic effect. For many patients it is their first opportunity to talk about their problems and cares. The interview alone can bring about a certain cathectic discharge immediately accompanied by a feeling of relief. The patient is then able to reconsider many issues in the absence of strong emotion. In addition to the advantages of this cathartic action, the patient has the impression of being understood for the first time and is given a chance of seeking a solution to his problems.

Before being given this initial opportunity of verbalizing their problems, the patients tended to brood day and night over them and consequently lacked objectivity. The doctors occasional questions are a further help to remedying this one-sided view of their problems, some of which are consciously perceived in their proper context for the first time.

The talk does not go to root of the actual conflict at this stage, but it can help patients to realize and clarify their conflicts. As solutions are brought nearer into view, the overall effect of the conversation may quite well lead to relieving the psychosomatic symptoms.

The doctor's advice during the talk also improves patient compliance with respect to taking medicaments prescribed. This is important since it appears that about one third of patients do not follow their doctor's instructions.

Supportive Therapy (Freyberger 1976)

This type of treatment centres mainly around building up a stable object relationship and promoting a sense of security by ego-strengthening and general encouragement.

It is a form of psychotherapy particularly suited to patients with severe physical and emotional disturbances. The aim here is not to disclose and work on conflicts but to afford support and promote a measure of autonomy. Helpful and reliable qualities on the part of the therapist are of particular importance in this type of therapy.

Individual Therapy

In order to apply this therapy successfully the patient must have motivation, emotional suffering and the ability to reflect on his own problems.

In its rather fixed setting of lying on a couch, free association and three to four attendances of one hour every week, psychoanalytical individual therapy assumes a large measure of tolerance to frustration, tension and anxiety on the part of the patient. In psychoanalytically orientated psychotherapy, which is characterized by a more active role on the part of the therapist and eye-to-eye contact, such requirements are not so rigorous. This type of psychotherapy is thus better suited to psychosomatic patients. The work here centres mainly around childhood key figures, relationship conflicts and transference.

Group Therapy

The collective treatment constituted by the group situation enables patients to obtain a picture of the workings of their minds and of their behaviour within a social framework. The group can provide a corrective emotional experience in a 'here and now' situation in that it affords the patients some protection against their innermost anxiety and some understanding of their needs. At the same time it can serve as a support and enhance their chances of coming to terms with reality.

The possible fragmentation of transference in the group tends to allay any fears of close personal proximity that may arise. If it is possible in the course of therapy to reintegrate such fragmented transference into the group as a whole, the needs of the patients regarding their own identity will be met.

This process often takes place in such a manner that typical, unconscious conflicts and patterns of interaction present themselves in 'scenes' (not necessarily explosive), after which they are brought clearer to light in the course of group work and that very part of his feelings that might be said to have become 'lost' becomes clearer to the patient.

Psychoanalytically orientated group therapy involves free association, as well as work on transference and resistance, with the therapist assuming the attitude of observer and participant alike. There are, however, other techniques of group therapy, the most important of which are interaction-process analysis, transactional analysis, psychodrama and Gestalt therapy.

Family Confrontation

Generally speaking, the psychosomatic patient is regarded in his milieu as being either a person with a serious organic illness, a trivial case, a hypochondriac or a malingerer (the opinions of close relatives fluctuate in a manner reminiscent of the variations of labile blood pressure and the opinions held!). Such fallacies only reinforce the symptoms and make the patient feel isolated and abandoned. A 'respectable' sickness status is accorded in the first instance to people with organic disorders, less to those with functional disturbances, and least of all to the emotionally ill and to psychosomatic patients. The latter are in fact subject to greater disrespect and injurious attitudes; being the socially and constitutionally weaker among their fellows, they are constrained to accept the type of patient role that society offers them. The plainly ill member of the family plays a similar role for the family unit as the neurotic situation does for the individual. The psychosomatic disorder of this individual is frequently a signal to the outside that something in the family as a unit is wrong (Pakesch 1974). We may thus speak of *family psychosomatics*.

We have consequently instituted a method of *confrontation with the family as an aid to therapy* (Gutter and Luban-Plozza 1978). The concept of family psychosomatics is not directed merely towards effecting a change for the better in the sick member but primarily towards improving intrafamilial relations. And this is precisely where the family doctor enjoys certain advantages. He is in a far better position than the specialist in that his knowledge of the patient goes beyond the mere case history since he has usually known the patient's family for some time, sometimes several generations of their history. Perhaps he is even acquainted with current family myths serving to justify or conceal painful realities in its history. This naturally facilitates his *entrée*.

Confrontation with the family is not identical with family therapy, although it paves the way for such treatment. The confrontation usually consists of a single, concentrated intervention. The talk should not exceed 30 to 60 minutes and may be held at the home of the family, at the surgery or in the hospital, depending on the doctor handling the case.

It is of considerable advantage when the doctor has already gained the confidence of the family member that has presented with symptoms. In this dialogue care should be taken not to interpret any connections between the patient's illness and the family constellation. This would only reinforce any existing feelings of guilt in the other members of the family and lead to further polarization between the sick member and the other 'healthy' members. The task of the doctor is to try and understand this focus, indicate the positive role the family can play and encourage a change in general behaviour. Such prompting of the family to enter into a constructive conversation on what can be done to make things easier, to change certain aspects, and provide help, has the long-term aim of restructuring the family constellation.

Family Therapy

According to Wirsching family therapy is indicated in cases where there are strong family ties involving mutual dependency among individual members, in severe psychosomatic crises and when the key patient has little motivation.

The psychosomatic patient is often the 'bearer of problems' for the entire family. In one respect, he constitutes a form of relief for the family since 'worrying' about him prevents the smouldering conflicts within the family from breaking out. In the long run, however, this sick member of the family brings added strain and uncertainty, also from the aspect of his presenting symptoms, which make his vexations and pathological conflicts apparent to outsiders.

It is often difficult to motivate the whole family to have a talk with the therapist. The symptom of their 'bearer of problems' that appears to afford so much relief for the rest of the family is accepted as 'permanent'. Its elimination would disturb a family equilibrium that has been maintained at the expense of so much trouble on their part, and cause the actual conflicts to break out.

Psychosomatic families have been described as closed systems with mutual dependency ties between the members, who are also under strong emotional pressures (Wirsching). Three prevailing modes of relationship in such families have been depicted by Stierlin in the following manner: The type of *bonding* that may delay or block the affected person's development in accordance with his age; *rejection*, which can lead to the patient neglecting his own person to the point of slovenliness, as well as to neglecting others in the sense of autistic withdrawal into himself, and exaggerated striving for autonomy. Finally, there is *delegation*, the pathological form of which is understood to be a family constellation, in which the parents, for example, ignore the true abilities of their children and press them into fulfilling their own unachieved ambitions.

According to Minuchin et al., interaction patterns in families afflicted with psychosomatic disturbances are characterized by involved situations and excessive solicitude, strict avoidance of conflict, stubbornness, and a tendency to trespass over generation boundaries.

Textor distinguishes between the following schools of family therapy largely by the types of treatment advocated, theoretical focus, and aim of therapy:

Strategic Family Therapy

Adherents of this trend are Haley, Jackson, Watzlawick and Weakland, Watzlawick et al., and the 'Milan school' (Selvini-Palazzoli et al.). They focus mainly on examining system processes as expressed in patterns of interaction, rules and behavioural facets. This school describes the sick families as rigidly balanced, closed systems with undefined relationships, fights for power, and bad communication between members. In a treatment comprising few sessions, the primary aim is to mitigate symptoms and resolve conflicts; problems are tackled one at a time and a fresh strategy is devised for each. In so doing, the therapists make wide and varied use of paradoxical methods, alter communicative behaviour and give 'homework'.

Structural Family Therapy
The principal advocates of this trend are Minuchin et al. They examine the relationship between the family and its milieu, the structure of familial subsystems (e.g grandparent-parent-child-generation), their limitations and the part each person plays in the system. According to this line of thought, sick families harbour intense marital conflict and are badly structured (coalitions across the generations, involved situations and excessive solicitude). The treatment consists in modifying the family structure and the part played by each. Techniques employed include modeling, observational learning, interpersonal accommodation, awareness training and interpretation.

Growth Orientated Family Therapy
Satir, Whitaker and Kempler are advocates of this trend. The therapeutic process focuses on each family member's affective experience, emotions, needs, and on the manner in which feelings are expressed. The symptom complex is explained by negative experiences and faulty communication. The treatment encourages members to acquire fresh experience of themselves and others, to accept both their own individual personality and that of fellow family members, and to become more spontaneous and independent. The therapists communicate their own feelings and experiences, behave naturally, and serve as model. Therapeutic techniques are also employed that relate to life situations such as psychodrama and sculpting.

Psychodynamic Family Therapy
Ackermann, Boszormenyi-Nagy and Sparke, Framo and Wynne favour this approach. They are primarily concerned with unconscious, intrapsychic and interpersonal processes, as well as with the development of the personality and the part played by each member. This school contends that symptoms occur on account of loyalty ties, transference entanglements, the according of roles, projections, myths and unconscious conflict. The treatment consists in examining the family development and life of each member, revealing the causes of conflicts, analyzing transference and resistance, and changing the course of familial and psychodynamic processes. Therapists employ interpretation, awareness training and confrontation. They endeavour to promote individuation and autonomy, stronger solidarity and better gratification of reciprocal requirements.

Petzold (1979) developed *family confrontation therapy* for the treatment of anorexia nervosa from the experience that strict separation of parents from patients proved of little value; it seemed as if the family's willingness to help must be brought to bear in a different manner.

One person alone cannot solve a family problem. It is thus necessary in family confrontation to make an intrafamilial approach to the trouble involved that enables all members to find a practical way out of their communication problems. The family therapy itself can then be commenced with a comprehensive diagnosis and possible solutions worked out.

During further development of the family confrontation therapy concept, certain elements of 'significant emotional experience' (Farrely and Brandsma; Whitaker) were integrated into the discussions held with families.

In anorexia nervosa, family therapy is supplemented by the formation of *parent groups*. These constitute for the parents involved a means of finding support during reverses and phases of despair. Parents also have the opportunity of recognizing and working through their own involvement in the illness and of finding alternatives to possibly rigid attitudes.

Parent groups may lend expression to the increasing individuation taking place in the presenting family member. Group work may bring some measure of relief to the family unit as a whole, which in turn tends to create more elbowroom in the presenting patient's life. Parent groups may also offer a framework within which intrafamilial shifts in symptoms such as depressive tendencies in a parent, or long-smouldering, hidden conflict, can be checked (Herzog et al.).

Psychosomatic Treatment in Hospital

Inpatient treatment makes it possible to employ simultaneous and supplementary procedures. As far as the patient is concerned, the artificial alternative between a somatic or psychic cause for the disorder then no longer exists [simultaneous diagnosis and therapy after Hahn (1988)]. Hospitalized psychosomatic treatment is indicated in obvious problem cases, all manner of crises, and for readmitted, decompensated chronically-ill patients with, say, Crohn's disease, ulcerative colitis, insulin-dependent diabetes or anorexia nervosa.

By virtue of its very location, psychosomatic treatment under hospitalization can have a lasting effect on reducing the crisis situation, so that a good point of departure is created for the final working through. Ideally, this should be family orientated and not carried out in a way that isolates the patient from an accustomed social context (Kröger et al. 1986; Bergmann et al. 1986). Inpatient treatment is, moreover, often indispensable for subsequent longterm outpatient therapy; only under hospitalized conditions are some patients able to gain insight into psychodynamic conflictual situations previously alien to them.

The hospital atmosphere is largely determined by the 'holding function' of the therapy team – a prime requirement for the supportive or uncovering/confronting techniques used. Depending on the therapeutic orientation followed, the choice lies between a wide range of individual and group therapies, usually supplemented by various forms of art therapy (painting, music, and dance) and relaxation techniques (autogenic training, functional relaxation, yoga, and meditation). All members of the therapy team exercise an integrative influence on the treatment process. This is important since disturbed communication and relationships can recur under hospitalized conditions. Such disturbances are discussed in team conferences and looked at in their entirety before targets are set and strategies developed.

Autogenic Training

Schultz developed autogenic training as a body therapy in which the patient learns relaxation and the lowering of muscle tone or vascular tension by regular practice of an autosuggestive technique. Employed individually or, preferably, in a group, it has proved of particular value as a 'psychosomatic bridging therapy'; while practising the technique, patients often experience for the first time the reciprocal influence of physical and mental processes.

Acquiring the ability of self-regulation by training affords support to autonomous needs, gives the patient the feeling he is doing something for his health and is responsible for it. 'Concentrated self-relaxation', as Schultz called his method, has been developed, or rather rediscovered, owing to the urgent needs of our time. If relaxation is beneficial, even essential, to healthy people, then it follows that it is even more essential to the large numbers of people suffering from functional disturbances. This method is widely used, particularly in the field of mental hygiene. The trained subject can acquire the ability to remain calm and collected, to recover his strength quickly and overcome sleep disturbances.

Psychosomatic Training

By psychosomatic training we understand a combination of exercises centred around breathing, which may in individual cases be supplemented by massage aimed at relaxation (Luban-Plozza, Basel).

Other body therapies include functional relaxation therapy and concentrative movement therapy. While self-awareness in the former is concentrated on feeling and sensation, movement therapy complements these events by the active experience of other group participants.

All three techniques are well suited to treating psychosomatic patients since they focus mainly on body sensations, body awareness and body image.

Supplementary Possibilities

Art therapy may make a useful contribution, but only if the patient really desires it, and it is not prescribed merely in order to keep him occupied. Such activity should be arranged with the idea in mind of giving the patient a means of re-establishing social relationships and stimulating his creative and imaginative impulses.

Functional disturbances respond well to physiotherapy, particularly in the form of breathing exercises, massage or baths. If the patient's attitude is too passive it can be rendered more active by gymnastics, or possibly by music and dance therapy. Much can be achieved if the patient is encouraged to apply self-help. It is first of all essential, however, that the doctor should explain – and that the patient should understand – exactly what each measure is designed to achieve.

The scope of multidimensional therapy (modified from Buser) is listed below:

- Medication and diet
- Physical therapy
- Mechanotherapy, orthopedic measures
- Climatotherapy
- Psychotherapy
- Psychopharmacotherapy
- Physiotherapy, especially breathing exercises, individual or group
- Occupational therapy in various forms, individual or group, developing actual rehabilitation
- Welfare services: family and marriage counseling, care of the elderly, advice in matters of finance and employment
- Spiritual (religious) support.

Prophylaxis

With more appreciation of the psychosocial factors responsible for the cause of illness, increased emphasis is rightly being placed on prevention. Considerations involving social conditions and mental health connected with the general way of life assume great importance; preventive medicine restricted to taking precautionary measures is too one-sided.

Here again, the best chances of contributing to prophylaxis in this sense are through the good offices of the general practitioner, who often has a more intimate knowledge of the emotional and social aspects of his patients' lives than either the specialist or members of other professions. Appeals have thus been made to physicians who do not limit their practice to a specialty to make a determined approach to such conflict situations. They can thus make valuable contributions to preventing behavioural disorders ending in psychosomatic symptoms. This is a wonderful opportunity to offer prophylactic aid to children at risk by exerting influence on the family as a whole.

It is indeed conceivable that guidance and care within the emotional constellation of the family will become a *foremost medical commitment*. Primary prophylaxis in mental hygiene is at the same time a social problem, an interdisciplinary problem. Doctors, psychologists, sociologists, theologists and teachers are thus involved in affording the ailing family the benefit of their specialized knowledge in order to give it new meaning.

12 Psychopharmacotherapy

The following sections deal with three groups of psychopharmaceuticals: antidepressants, tranquilizers ('minor tranquilizers'), and neuroleptics ('major tranquilizers').

Problems involving stimulants, nootropics and hypnotics in toto are excluded.

12.1 Antidepressants

After all the disputes concerning the antidepressant effect of benzodiazepine derivatives, the main requirements for an antidepressant remain as follows: The drug may be so termed provided it is capable of satisfactorily elevating mood during endogenous depression in a patient known to suffer from a manic-depressive illness. A further criterion is that this should occur within the first three months of the phase since spontaneous remission is also possible. The discussion as to whether benzodiazepines exert also an antidepressant action arose since depressive states mostly go hand in hand with anxiety, which can additionally be treated with benzodiazepine derivates. Should benzodiazepines be used alone, however, the patient may indeed feel much better after taking the first and each subsequent dose, but the treatment does not constitute real improvement in the sense of elevating depressed mood.

When antidepressants are prescribed, patients should be told they may initially experience such side effects as tiredness, more need for sleep, inner unrest, increased dream activity, palpitation, sweating, and accommodative disturbances, but that these will recede after a few days. A slow, mood-brightening effect then usually sets in. In this case, relief does not occur after each dose, but a gradual elevation of mood takes place over the entire course of the treatment.

The situation is quite different in cases of nonendogenous and particularly of mild depression, where, for example, the reactive variety of the illness can readily be treated with benzodiazepines or neuroleptics, which may then become unnecessary after a few days.

Non-MAO inhibitor antidepressants have the following mechanism of action: In phase 1 the re-uptake inhibitors (see Fig. 12) lead to an inhibition

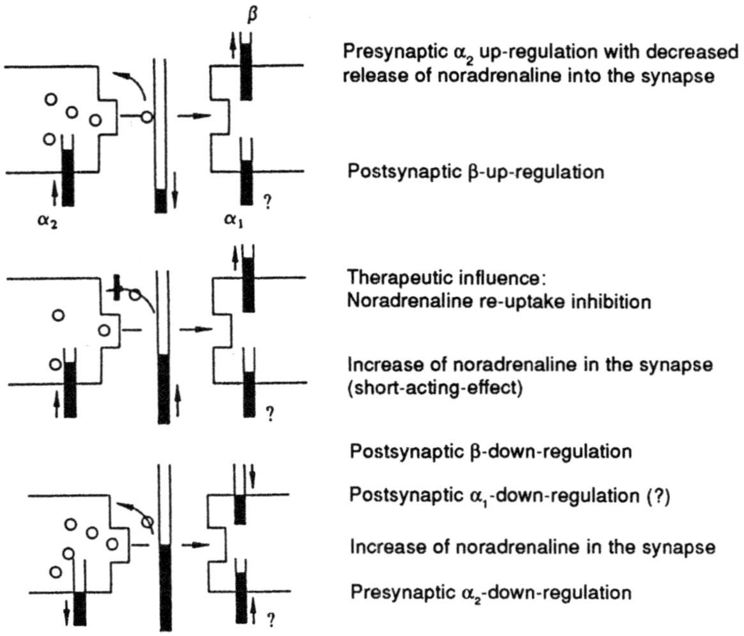

Fig. 12. Synaptic processes in depression

of the re-uptake of biogenic amines in the presynaptic cleft, where raised concentrations of them consequently occur. (MAO inhibitors block the breakdown of biogenic amines at this location). Research has so far shown these biogenic amines to be depleted in cases of depression. In phase 2 (relating to the long-acting effect) there is a reduction in postsynaptic sensitivity. This is particularly true of β-receptors, and also of serotonergic receptors in the sense of competitive action. The degree and extent to which the various neurotransmitters are affected during these processes is determined by the type of antidepressant prescribed.

Table 10 gives a breakdown of this action on transmitter substances by various antidepressants. The question arises whether individual concentrations play a role, or whether, as assumed relatively early by Riederer and Birkmayer, the concentrations of the various transmitter substances relative to one another are more important.

Based on the schema drawn up by Kielholz et al. (1981), Table 11 collates antidepressants in use today in accordance with their psychomotor activating, stabilizing and sedating properties. As far as re-uptake inhibitors are concerned, a difference exists between tricyclic and nontricyclic antidepressants in that the nontricyclic are generally better tolerated with respect to autonomic and cardiac side effects, while the classic tricyclic antidepressants bring about the desired action more frequently and effectively. In this connection, the slow reduction of postsynaptic receptor sen-

Table 10. A classification of antidepressants according to their biochemical properties. (Abridged and modified from Gastpar 1980)

INN	NE	SE	DA	H_1	Ach	$5\text{-}HT_2$
Desipramine	+	–	–	–	+	
Imipramine	+	(+)	–	+	+	
Maprotiline	+	–	–	+	(+)	(+)
Fluvoxamine	–	+	–	–	–	
Trazodone	(+)	+	–	–	–	+
Mianserin	+	–	–		(+)	+
Amitriptyline	(+)	+	–	+	+	+
Trimipramine	–	–	–	+	+	

NE, inhibition of noradrenaline uptake.
SE, inhibition of serotonin uptake.
DA, activation of dopaminergic neurons.
H_1, action on histamine$_1$ receptors.
Ach, anticholinergic action.
$5\text{-}HT_2$, action on serotonin$_2$ receptors.

Table 11. A classification of antidepressants (after Kielholz)

		Psychomotor activating	Psychomotor stabilizing	Psychomotor sedating
Non-MAO inhibitors	Tricyclics	Desipramine Nortriptyline Protriptyline	Imipramine Chlomipramine Melitracen Dimetacrine Noxiptiline Lofepramine	Amitriptyline Amitriptilinoxide Trimipramine Doxepine Dosulepin Butriptyline
	Nontricyclics		Maprotiline Mianserin Viloxazin Fluvoxamine	Trazodone
	Precursors			L-Tryptophan Tryptophan Oxitriptan
MAO-inhibitors		Isocarboxazide Tranylcypromine		

sitivity appears to play a special role, for this does not only occur in treatment with re-uptake inhibitors but also in that carried out with MAO inhibitors, in sleep deprivation and electroconvulsive therapy.

Since the mood-elevating effect of antidepressant therapy occurs only after some days have elapsed, this period must be bridged in serious cases by simultaneous administration of a neuroleptic or benzodiazepine preparation, which is discontinued when the antidepressant takes effect. Among this category are patients with suicidal tendencies, intense anxiety and agitation, or severe sleep disturbances.

Carbamazepine, originally an anticonvulsant, is acquiring increased importance in treating dysphoric, depressive, and particularly rapid, mood changes ('rapid cycler'). In addition to these relatively new indications, carbamazepine, like lithium salts, has proved of value as prophylaxis against manic-depressive relapse. An analogous development is seen with valproic acid.

12.2 Neuroleptics

In common with all the modern tranquilizers, neuroleptics may be defined as having a sleep-inducing rather than a hypnotic action. In addition, however, this group of psychopharmaceuticals has been shown to have certain effects on schizophrenic illnesses, acting against thought disorders, delusions, hallucinations, and some negative symptoms, which in their extreme form constitute autism. Besides their sedative property, neuroleptics have been shown experimentally to have a cataleptic effect, inhibit certain reflexes, have antiemetic and adrenolytic actions, and potentiate the effects of alcohol, barbiturates, and opium alkaloids. They are, however, antagonistic to the excitatory effect of amphetamines. Certain neuroleptics exhibit a convulsant action; they lower the convulsive threshold compared with pentylentetrazol and electroshock. They also blockade dopamine, noradrenaline, and serotonin receptors in the central synapses. From an electrophysiological point of view the reticular formation is screened against external stimuli (see Fig. 13). Thus, the arousal reaction of the reticular activating system on the cortex, and even on endocrinological and autonomic centres, is naturally inhibited.

Figure 14 sets out various neuroleptics in relation to their spectrum of activity (after Lambert and Calanca 1988). It shows that neuroleptics active in high doses have primarily sedative properties, while those tending to be active in low doses possess a more marked 'antipsychotic' action, i.e. against schizophrenic thought disorders, delusions, illusions and hallucinations. Those preparations prescribed in particularly small doses act not only antipsychotic but also antiautistic.

The depot and retard preparations listed in Table 12 are important, particularly for schizophrenic patients, who have a frequent tendency to discontinue medication on discharge. They consider themselves healthy again and it is then very difficult to get them to resume taking the drug prescribed. All too often this results in further hospitalization. This revolving-door phenomenon could be effectively countered by employing depot

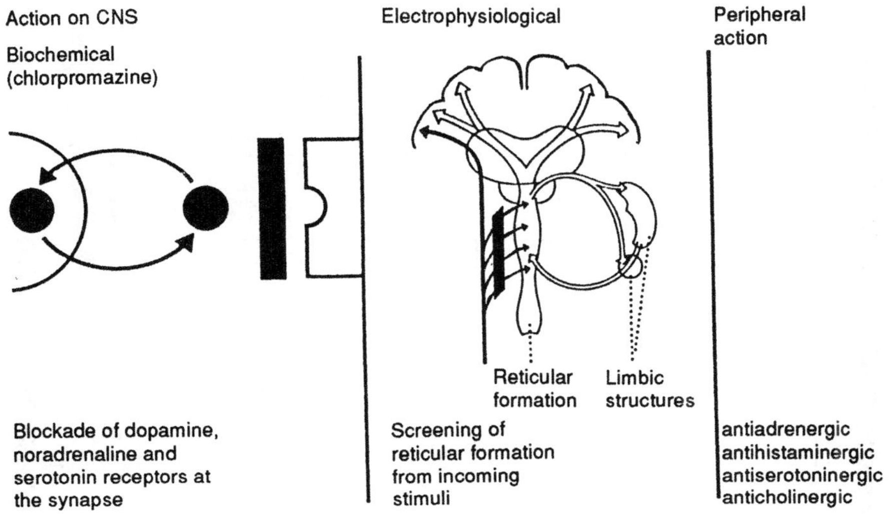

Fig. 13. Mechanisms of action in treatment with neuroleptics

neuroleptics injected every two to three weeks. Despite the slow release of active substance, marked sedation usually occurs shortly after the injection, which patients tend to fear. This situation can be prevented by oral doses of neuroleptic over a few days prior to the repeat depot injection. During this period the effect of the previous injection is already diminishing and, by virtue of the additional doses per os, the sedative action of the next will not be experienced so abruptly.

It is important, especially in chronic schizophrenia, to commence with a programme of rehabilitation that is socially as well as psychiatrically orientated, so that the patient can be reintegrated into family and working life as soon as possible. The general practitioner has an important part to play during this phase, particularly with respect to the timely and regular administration of the depot neuroleptic. Should the injection become considerably overdue, it is then extremely difficult in most cases to convince the patient of the necessity to continue therapy. Here again, we see this repeatedly result in relapse and further hospitalization.

12.3 Tranquilizers

This third group of psychopharmaceuticals comprises what are sometimes called the 'minor tranquilizers', 90% of which are now benzodiazepine derivatives. The pros and cons of these substances have been widely dis-

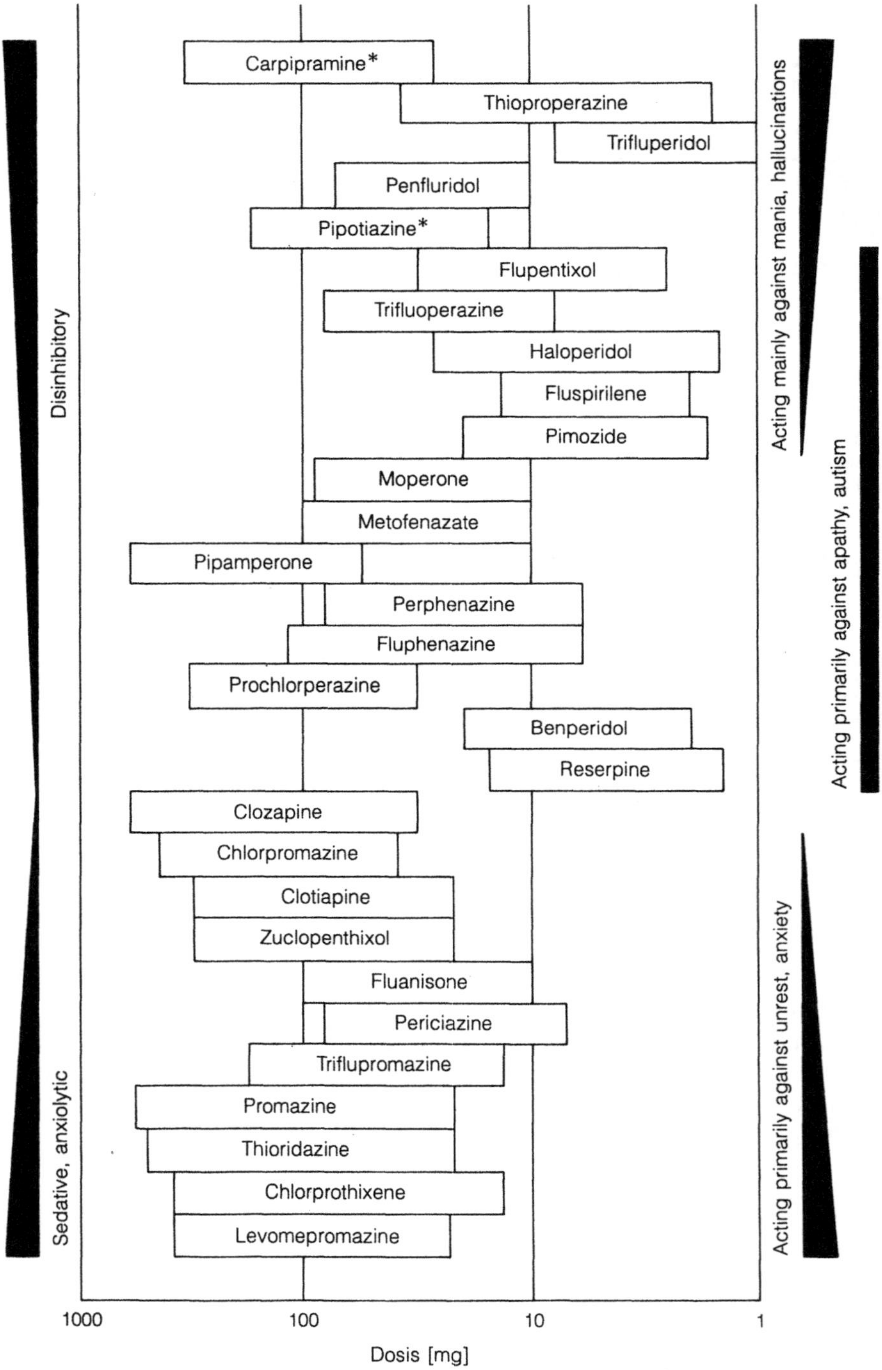

Fig. 14. The dosage range for various neuroleptic drugs (nonproprietary names). (Modified after Lambert and Revol 1960; Calanca 1988)

Table 12. Depot and retard neuroleptics (after Pöldinger 1982)

Generic name	Brand name	Route of administration	Average dose (mg)	Duration of action
Depot				
Fluphenazine decanoate	Dapotum D	i.m.	12.5–100	2–3 weeks
	Modecate			
	Anatensol			
	Prolixin			
Perphenazine denanthate	Decentan Depot	i.m.	100	1–2 weeks
	Fentazin			
Pipotiazine palmitate	Piportil Depot	i.m.	75	4 weeks
Flupentixol decanoate	Fluanxol Depot	i.m.	20–60	2–4 weeks
	Depixol			
Zuclopenthixol acetate	Clopixol Acutard	i.m.	50–150	3 days
Zuclopenthixol decanoate	Cisordinol Depot	i.m.		
	Clopixol Depot			
Haloperidol decanoate	Haldol Decanoate	i.m.	50–200	4 weeks
Fluspirilene	Imap	i.m.	2–6	1 week
	Redeptin			
Penfluridol	Semap	p.o.	10–40 (60)	1 week
Retard				
Thioridazine	Melleril 30 retard	p.o.	60–600	24 h
Fluphenazine 2HCL*	Lyogen retard	p.o.	1–2 ret. drg.	24 h
	Moditen; Anatensol			
Moperone	Luvatren retard	p.o.	20–40	24 h
Pimozide	Orap	p.o.	2–6	24 h
Bromperidol	Impromen	p.o.	1–6	24 h
	Tesoprel	i.m., iv.		

* All forms of fluphenazine dihydrochloride have an intrinsic 24-hour action.

Table 13. The polarization of pharmacotherapy

Relief of anxiety (anxiolytic effects)	Activation of anxiety
Tranquilizers	Centrally acting stimulants
Neuroleptics	Appetite depressants
Antidepressants with anxiolytic components	Antidepressants with activating properties
Sedatives	Psycholytics
Hypnotics	
β-adrenergic blocking agents	
Opiates	
Bromides	

Table 14. Important pharmacological actions and their use in treatment (after Haefely 1980)

Pharmacological actions	Clinical indications
Anxiolytic, acting against conflict and frustration	Anxiety, phobia Anxiety depression
Disinhibition of certain forms of behaviour	Neurotic inhibitions
Anticonvulsant	The most varying types of epileptiform activity (epilepsy, convulsive poisoning)
Inhibition of readiness for psychical reaction to stimuli (sedation)	Hyperemotional states Schizophrenia (?)
Sleep-inducing action	Sleep disorders
Inhibition of centrally transmitted autonomic response to emotional and psychic stimuli	Psychosomatic disorders (cardiovascular, gastrointestinal, urogenital, hormonal)
Central lowering of skeletal muscle tone	Muscular spasm of somatic or psychogenic origin, tetanus
Reinforces action of centrally acting drugs, anterograde amnesia	Anesthetic for surgical and diagnostic interventions
No direct action outside the central nervous system Exceptionally low toxicity	

cussed, a popular mistake being to associate benzodiazepines fully with the term anxiolytics since part of their action is to reduce anxiety. Table 13 lists two groups of drugs with opposing effects.

Table 14, modified from Haefely (1980), shows which pharmacological properties correspond to certain clinical actions. It thus illustrates the applicational range of benzodiazepines in either hospitals or general practice.

An interesting aspect concerning the mechanism of action of these substances has been the discovery of benzodiazepine receptors in the brain.

Table 15. Tranquilizers

Generic name	Generic name
1. Anxiolytic tranquilizers	2. Other tranquilizers
Benzodiazepine derivatives	
Alprazolam	Buspiron
Bromazepam	Clomethiazol
Camazepam	Methylpentynol
Chlordiazepoxide	Trimetozine
Clobazam	
Clorazepate Dipotassium	3. Benzodiazepine antagonists
Clotiazepam	
Cloxazolam	Flumazenil
Delorazepam	
Diazapam	4. Sleep inducing tranquilizers
Ketazolam	
Lorazepam	Benzodiazepine derivatives
Medazepam	
Metaclazepam	Brotizolam
Nordazepam	Flunitrazepam
Oxazepam	Flurazepam
Oxazolam	Laprozolam
Prazepam	Lormetazepam
	Midazolam
Dibenzobicyclo-octadiene derivatives	Nitrazepam
Benzoctamine	Temazepam
	Triazolam
Diphenylmethane derivatives	
Hydroxyzine	
Propranediol derivatives	
Mebrobamate	

These receptors work very closely together with those for GABA (γ-aminobutyric acid). They are assigned primarily to the reciprocally inhibiting neurons.

Benzodiazepine derivatives, whether prescribed as daytime tranquilizers or as hypnotics, produce rebound effects. Habituation and dependence are also possible, and though substance dependence is rare, a certain addictive potential has on occasion been observed. This aspect is dealt with later in the section on concomitant effects. In Table 15, tranquilizers at present available are listed systematically according to their principal foci of action. It will be seen that there is a considerable variety of benzodiazepine derivatives on the market, many having specific indications. Although their mode of action is in principle the same, according to dosage they can be recommended either as daytime tranquilizers or as hypnotics. Short-acting benzodiazepines are now mainly the drugs of choice for sleep disturbances.

All preparations belonging to this class in the widest sense should ideally be prescribed as part of a general strategy centred around psychotherapy.

The plan must be discussed in detail with all patients individually. They should be informed not only of the positive results expected but also of possible unwanted effects.

12.4 Concomitant Effects

As it has not yet been established whether several of the so-called side effects of psychopharmaceuticals are in fact side effects or are not just closely related to the psychotropic action, we prefer to use the term concomitant effects. The most important of these effects are shown in Table 16.

12.4.1 Neuroleptics

The prolonged use of *neuroleptics* leads in particular to *extrapyramidal symptoms* ranging from tremor to a fully-fledged Parkinson's syndrome. Neuroleptics – especially those with no initial sleep-inducing effect – can produce during the first few days or weeks of treatment painful paroxysmal muscle spasm (dyskinesia) particularly in the muscles of the mouth, tongue and pharynx. Antiparkinsonian agents, if necessary administered i.v. or i.m., have proved effective in the treatment of these phenomena.

The use of neuroleptics over a period of years can result in *tardive dyskinesia*, which, unlike the dyskinesia that occurs during the initial stages of therapy, is little influenced by antiparkinsonian agents and, like autonomic symptoms, can be induced or aggravated by the sudden withdrawal of the neuroleptic. However, since persistent dyskinesia of this type occurs only rarely (shown by our investigations in two psychiatric hospitals) and can also be due to factors other than drugs, it must be accepted as a therapeutic risk; nevertheless we feel constrained to lay down particularly strict limits to the indications of long-term therapy with neuroleptics. If this type of dyskinesia occurs as a result of sudden withdrawal of neuroleptics it can be eliminated or greatly alleviated by recommencing administration of the drug.

12.4.2 Antidepressants

Antidepressants are associated mainly with *autonomic concomitant effects*, usually of an adrenergic type. These can be relieved with adrenolytics such as co-dergocrine-mesylate (<Hydergine>). As is to be expected on the basis of the pharmacological data alone, neuroleptics can also produce autonomic symptoms, whereas these do not occur in the case of treatment with tranquilizers.

Table 16. The principal concomitant effects and complications of psychopharmaceuticals

	Neuroleptics	Tranquilizers	Thymoleptics	MAO inhibitors
Neurological concomitant effects	Tremor, parkinsonism, dyskinesia	Innervation disturbances	Tremor	
Autonomic concomitant effects	Orthostatic hypotension, sweating, dizziness		Dryness of mouth, tachycardia, sweating, dizziness, micturition disturbances	Orthostatic hypotension, possibility of hypertonic crises
General condition	Fatigue		Fatigue, inner restlessness	
Psychopathological concomitant effects	Transitory paradoxical states of agitation	Habituation	Delirious states Swing to hypomanic phase, activation of acute schizophrenic symptoms	
Dangerous combinations	Potentiation of the effects of alcohol and barbiturates		Incompatibility with MAO inhibitors	Incompatibility with thymoleptics and cheese

The most important of the *psychopathological complications* are the transient paradoxical states of agitation produced by neuroleptics and the induction of acute schizophrenic or manic symptoms together with the appearance of transient delirious states resulting from the administration of antidepressants. When prescribing psychopharmaceuticals it should also be borne in mind that thymoleptics are incompatible with monoamine oxidase inhibitors and that monoamine oxidase inhibitors are incompatible with cheese; patients should be warned of the possible impairment of behaviour in traffic and of the potentiation of the effects of alcohol.

12.4.3 Tranquilizers

It has already been pointed out that 'rebound phenomena' may arise in the wake of benzodiazepine therapy. In this context, the term relates to recurrence of prior symptoms after medication is discontinued. It is easy to confuse the rebound phenomenon with the original symptom complex, wrongly conclude that medication should be resumed, and even that the dosage be increased.

Benzodiazepine derivatives have a certain addictive potential; habituation and dependence, and in rare cases substance dependence, have been encountered. Treatment with these drugs should thus be as short as possible. It is far too little known that rebound phenomena can be avoided by

Table 17. β-adrenergic blocking agents: CNS

Anxiety:	
Anxiety attack	+++
Generalized anxiety	
with physical symptoms	+++
without physical symptoms	?
Anxiety in depression	++
Psychosomatic disorders	
with cardiovascular involvement	+++
without cardiovascular involvement	?
Examination anxiety and stage fright	
with physical symptoms	++
Phobias	(+)
Stuttering	+
Tremor:	
Lithium-type	++
Essential	+
Alcoholic	+
Parkinsonism	(+)
Tardive dyskinesia and akathisia	+
Withdrawal symptoms	+
Migraine (regular)	++
Psychoses:	
Prophyria	(+)
Schizophrenia	(+)
Mania	(+)

discontinuing medication gradually and not abruptly. This can be done along the following lines: One tablet three times daily, for example, may initially be reduced by a quarter of a tablet, then lowered further at about weekly intervals. If the symptoms call for it, the dosage should provisionally be retained before further attempts at reduction are made. Severe cases of benzodiazepine dependence can often be resolved only over weeks or even months. When unpleasant disorders, especially autonomic, occur during this phase, β-blockers can prove of value.

Patients susceptible to the abuse of alcohol, hypnotics and analgesics should be excluded from benzodiazepine treatment and be prescribed small doses of neuroleptics or antidepressants. Moreover, β-adrenergic blocking agents are gaining ground in the tranquilizer range of indications. The most important psychiatric and neurological indications for β-blockers are shown in Table 17.

Particularly with the elderly, care must be taken that the muscle relaxant properties of tranquilizers do not lead to disturbances in innervation and bring about eventual collapse.

12.5 Intoxication with Psychopharmaceuticals

Since psychopharmaceuticals, in particular antidepressants, are frequently prescribed for suicidal patients, it is obvious that drugs intended by the doctor as treatment will often be used by such patients with suicidal intent. It should be pointed out from the outset that, with the exception of the tricyclic antidepressants, patients have survived the ingestion of amazingly large quantities of neuroleptics and tranquilizers without any serious complications. Loew has summarized the study of patients admitted to our hospital following suicide attempts with psychopharmaceuticals. The highest doses survived without any permanent complications were 5,000 mg for neuroleptics such as chlorpromazine, 1,250 mg for antidepressants such as imipramine and 250 mg for tranquilizers such as benzodiazepine derivatives. Considerably higher doses have been reported in the world literature.

We have already said that tricyclic antidepressants constituted an anomaly in this respect. These are particularly toxic in small children, a few tablets accidentally consumed by a child often being sufficient to cause death. It is therefore imperative for doctors to impress upon patients for whom they prescribe tricyclic antidepressants or any other type of drug that they must keep them out of the reach of small children. When the drugs are no longer needed they should not be stored, nor should they be thrown into the dustbin, where they are not always safe from children, but they should be destroyed in some other way. Whereas even relatively high doses of neuroleptics usually produce only drowsiness or loss of consciousness, possibly accompanied by a tendency to collapse, and tranquilizers cause mainly relaxation of the peripheral skeletal muscles, tricyclic antidepressants can produce series of epileptic seizures and severe cardiac arrhythmias with bizarre effects in the ECG.

If one attempts to summarize the results of the Basle Symposium on the treatment of acute intoxications with psychopharmaceuticals then one could say that in general the so-called Scandinavian method after Clemmesen has proved its worth, although with a number of modifications:

1. In contrast to barbiturate intoxication, evacuation of the stomach may be indicated in overdosage of psychopharmaceuticals. Antidepressants especially inhibit peristalsis and thus prolong the length of time the drug remains in the stomach. Gastric lavage should, however, be carried out in unconscious patients only in conjunction with an endotracheal catheter and inflated balloon to prevent aspiration.
2. The first measure in collapse is not administration of cardiocirculatory agents, but, especially in intoxication with antidepressants, of blood substitutes and blood. If this is not effective, an infusion of angiotensin should be begun. Norepinephrine may be given only very cautiously by infusion, which is easily controllable. Since tricyclic antidepressants sensitize peripheral synapses to norepinephrine and monoamine oxidase inhibitors counter the breakdown of norepinephrine, administration of norepinephrine in the event of collapse can give rise to hypertensive crises, possibly leading to cerebral hemorrhage and death.
3. In hypertensive crises phentolamine or neuroleptics such as chlorpromazine can be tried.
4. In respiratory depression: artificial respiration without analeptics.
5. In epileptoid seizures and excitation: anticonvulsants i.v. and i.m., possibly small doses of neuroleptics or diazepam. (*Caution*: The effect of barbiturates is potentiated by many psychopharmaceuticals).
6. On disturbance of conduction or initiation of the heartbeat: not quinidine, but cardiotonics or pyridostigmine.
7. In dyskinesia or other extrapyramidal disturbances: antiparkinsonian agents i.v. or i.m.
8. Osmotic and saluretic dialysis is not known to be as effective in intoxication due to psychopharmaceuticals as in that due to barbiturates.

12.6 When Psychopharmaceuticals are Indicated in Psychosomatic Illness

Autonomic disturbances occur as concomitant symptoms in psychogenic and endogenous mental disorders but may also be precursors of such disorders or general irritation phenomena. They involve predominantly the peripheral autonomic nervous system and consequently are often treated with peripherally acting drugs.

However, our experience has shown that psychopharmaceuticals are superior in these disorders too, since we are not dealing purely and simply with an adrenergic or cholinergic deviation but rather with a state of dysregulation or lability.

Psychopharmaceuticals are also indicated in the treatment of psychosomatic disorders in the narrow sense. However, it is important to remember here that even in this type of pathological process psychopharmaceuticals do not themselves have any actual causal effect; instead they merely play a supportive role in that they prepare the patient for psychotherapy or render him accessible to it. In many cases psychopharmaceuticals will also help to bridge the gap before the aid of a psychotherapist can be enlisted. Naturally, treatment of these psychosomatic disorders must be carried out on two levels in that intensive somatotherapy must be implemented, a rule that also applies to psychotherapy. The problems involved in autonomic function, the disorders with which they are associated, and the relevant pharmacotherapy have figured in a publication by Labhardt (1970).

12.7 Chronic Pain

It has been shown, particularly in the chronic pain due to metastatic carcinoma, that neuroleptics not only allow the dose of morphine otherwise prescribed to be reduced but also that it is possible in many cases to obtain considerable relief by the use of neuroleptics alone. It is also possible to reduce consumption of analgesics by means of antidepressants, and even a combination neuroleptics and antidepressants is often suitable. One could perhaps liken the effect of neuroleptics in chronic pain to the result of prefrontal lobotomy. It is so to speak not the peripheral perception of pain but the mental processing of pain in the central nervous system, the actual experience of pain, that is affected.

In this context we should also mention the modern technique of neuroleptanalgesia used in anesthesiology; highly effective analgesics are combined with potent neuroleptics to permit painful operations to be carried out on conscious patients. This is of particular value in operations requiring the cooperation of the patient for the purpose of testing functions, for example, in the field of neurosurgery.

12.8 Suicidal Tendencies

Disorders with depressive overtones, especially when combined with anxiety, are associated with increased risk of suicide. It is therefore important when prescribing psychopharmaceuticals to bear in mind their effect in this regard. Of significance is that antidepressants exert their effect in the main only after several days or even weeks. In cases where there is a high suicide risk it is necessary to commence treatment with combined antidepressant and neuroleptic therapy. Neuroleptics help in reducing suicidal tendencies initially, and may be discontinued when the patient begins to respond to the antidepressant. In cases where the risk is less grave and it is desired to restrict medication to one drug, it is advisable to select an antidepressant with a sedative effect and prescribe the main dose for the evening. Disinhibiting antidepressants can initially increase anxiety and thus suicidal tendencies.

In order for suicidal tendencies to be treated they must first be recognized for what they are. Various methods have been formulated to assess the risk, but we should first like to mention Ringel's (1969a,b) presuicidal syndrome, which describes the dynamics involved in the development of the suicidal impulse. This may be employed by nonspecialists and even lay people, whereas another method, developed by Mitterauer and known as the 'suicidal axis syndrome', is more for the physician and psychiatrist.

Further pointers have been supplied by Kielholz, who classified factors contributing to the assessment of suicidal impulses in depressive patients.

The Presuicidal Syndrome (after Ringel)

1. Growing sense of constriction:
   (a) situational constriction;
   (b) psychodynamic constriction (narrowing of apperception, associations, behaviour patterns, emotions and defence mechanisms);
   (c) limitation of interpersonal relationships;
   (d) narrowing sense of values.
2. Pent-up or inturned aggression.
3. Suicidal fantasies (at first deliberately conjured up, later intruding involuntarily).

The Suicidal Axis Syndrome (after Mitterauer)

1. Overt or covert suicidal tendencies.
2. Diagnosis of an endomorphic-cyclothymic, endomorphic-schizophrenic and/or organic axis syndrome.
3. Positive evidence of suicide in the family history.

Assessment of Suicidal Tendencies (after Kielholz and Compiled in Accordance with Im Obersteg, Ringel, Stengel)

A. Direct evidence and pointers
1. Earlier suicide attempts or indications of suicidal bent.
2. Incidence of suicide in the family or environment (suggestive element).
3. Explicit or implicit suicide threats.
4. Direct reference to mode of execution of or preparations for suicide.

5. An ‘ominous calm’ following expression of suicidal intentions and state of unrest.
6. Dreams of self-destruction, downfall and catastrophe.

B. Special symptoms and syndromes
1. Anxiety and agitation.
2. Chronic sleep disturbances.
3. Pent-up emotion and aggression.
4. Onset or end of depressive phase, mixed states.
5. Periods of biological crisis (puberty, pregnancy, puerperium, menopause).
6. Strong feelings of guilt and inadequacy.
7. Incurable disease.
8. Hypochondriasis.
9. Alcoholism or drug addiction.

C. Environmental factors
1. Broken home in childhood.
2. Lack or loss of interpersonal contacts (isolation, uprooting, unhappy love affair).
3. Professional or financial problems.
4. Lack of a task or aim in life.
5. Lack or loss of sustaining religious beliefs.

Finally, we have the questionnaire for assessing suicidal tendencies formulated by Pöldinger. As these tendencies can undergo rapid change and their assessment is difficult, a compilation of all risk factors has but limited value. Nor have attempts to quantify such information been very successful. For this reason the items comprising the Pöldinger questionnaire have been restricted solely to those considered important for a direct assessment of the individual suicide risk.

Questionnaire for Assessing Suicidal Tendencies (after Pöldinger and Wider 1986):
The more questions 1–11 are answered with ‘yes’ and 12–16 with ‘no’, the greater is the risk of suicide.

1. Have you thought of taking your own life recently? Yes
2. Often? Yes
3. Have you had to think of it without wanting to?
   Do such suicide thoughts force themselves upon you? Yes
4. Do you have precise ideas how you would do it? Yes
5. Have you made preparations? Yes
6. Have you spoken to anyone about your suicidal intentions? Yes
7. Have you ever tried to commit suicide? Yes

8.	Has anyone in your family or among your friends and acquaintances ever committed suicide?	Yes
9.	Do you consider your situation desperate or hopeless?	Yes
10.	Do you have difficulty thinking about matters other than your problems?	Yes
11.	Have you had less contact with family, friends and acquaintances in recent times?	Yes
12.	Are you still interested in what goes on around you or in your work? Are you still interested in your hobbies?	No
13.	Do you have anyone with whom you can speak freely and in confidence about your problems?	No
14.	Do you live with someone else, for instance family or friends?	No
15.	Do you feel you have strong family or professional responsibilities?	No
16.	Do you feel you have roots in a religious or ideological community?	No
	Number of questions answered as in answer column	___
	Maximum	16

12.9 Drug Abuse and the Suicidal Impulse

In addition to acute intoxications, psychopharmaceuticals in the narrow sense, such as neuroleptics, tranquilizers and antidepressants, and also other drugs that act on the central nervous system, have other close associations with suicide. It is not without good reason that drug dependency has been described as a 'protracted form of suicide'. In our hospital, Battegay and Kielholz in particular have pointed out these close associations. Our own investigation in 440 patients admitted to hospital after suicide attempts showed 8% to be dependent on drugs and 9% to be alcoholics, i.e. an addiction rate of 17%. Next to depression of varying etiology, which accounted for 49%, and psychopathic personalities, which accounted for 18%, this is therefore the third largest diagnostic group with suicidal tendencies. However, as shown by Battegay and Kielholz, where the latent self-destructive impulses associated with addiction are concerned, the disturbed personality development is a more crucial factor than the chemical nature of the drug involved. Edwards holds a similar opinion: 'In essence what all statistical findings and dynamic insights point to is the fact that in studying addiction we should not make our focus the drug but the person and the person's setting.'

It is extremely difficult to determine whether the psychopharmaceuticals in the narrow sense lead simply to abuse or whether they can lead to actual addiction. One of the investigations carried out by Battegay at the Basle Hospital showed that sudden withdrawal of neuroleptics and antidepressants after a long period of treatment produces withdrawal symptoms such as

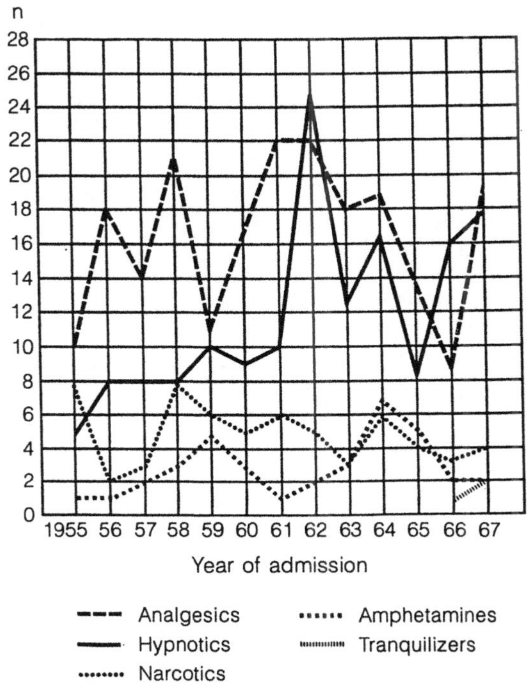

Fig. 15. Principal addictive agents: first admissions due to drug abuse

nausea, vomiting, sweating, collapse and extrapyramidal symptoms. This thus fulfils one of the criteria of addiction laid down by the WHO, namely physical dependence, even though these patients did not at the same time exhibit emotional dependence or increased tolerance. Battegay therefore raised the question of whether, in the light of these findings, the definition of addiction ought not to be revised.

Whilst as yet practically no cases of abuse of neuroleptics and antidepressants have been reported there have been occasional instances involving tranquilizers. Nevertheless it must be stressed that by comparison with the widespread use of these preparations the reports refer to only isolated cases. On the other hand, however, the turnover in these drugs shows that they are not taken or even prescribed for strictly medical indications only. This is borne out in an investigation by Kranz.

Figure 15 shows the first admissions of patients to the Psychiatric Clinic of Basle University Hospital on account of drug abuse or dependence between the years 1955 and 1967. It can be seen from this that, compared with the other groups of drugs, tranquilizers played a minor role.

This was also revealed by a Swiss Federal inquiry into the incidence of drug abuse carried out by Kielholz (1967, 1968). In this investigation a risk factor was calculated by correlating the number of tablets sold in Switzerland

Table 18. Time span between the introduction of a preparation and the first report of its abuse

Drug	Year of introduction	Year of the first publication on abuse	Authors	Difference in years
Analgesic combination (<Saridon>)	1933	1948	Jasinski, Fahrni	15
Glutethimide (<Doriden>)	1955	1957	Battegay	2
Methyprylon (<Noludar>)	1955	1960	Jensen	5
Meprobamate (<Miltown> and others)	1955	1956	Lemere	1
Chlordiazepoxide (<Librium>)	1961	1963	Guile	2
Diazepam (<Valium> Roche)	1963	1964	Lingjaerde	1

with the number of cases of abuse recorded by the investigation. The risk factor for analgesics was set at 1. The corresponding risk factor for hypnotics was 2.7 and for central stimulants 3.8 but for all the tranquilizers on the market the risk factor was only 0.2.

However, it is those very tranquilizers that show that the relationships between the pharmacogenic effect on the one hand and the psychodynamic process on the other still remain to be fully clarified. For if there were a closer correlation between addictive personality and potential risk of addiction to a drug, the highest incidence of abuse should occur with the drugs for which suspected abuse was reported quite shortly after their introduction (see Table 18). However, Fig. 16 shows that this is not so; it shows the difference in years between introduction and the first reports of abuse, and sets this against the first admissions of established cases of abuse at the Basle Psychiatric Hospital between 1962 and 1964.

It can be seen from this that for those drugs where the possibility of abuse had been reported shortly after their introduction, the actual number of confirmed cases of abuse is very small, while for an analgesic combination that had already been subject to frequent abuse by hospitalized patients fifteen years had elapsed before the first cases of abuse were reported. With respect to suicide prophylaxis, too, this means that the type of drug abused permits no conclusions to be drawn about the suicide risk, and that therapy must be conceived less in terms of the drug – for example in the withdrawal phase – and far more in terms of the personality of the patient.

Finally, we must mention the special case of lysergic acid diethylamide (LSD) and other psycholytics, which even if only because of the marked

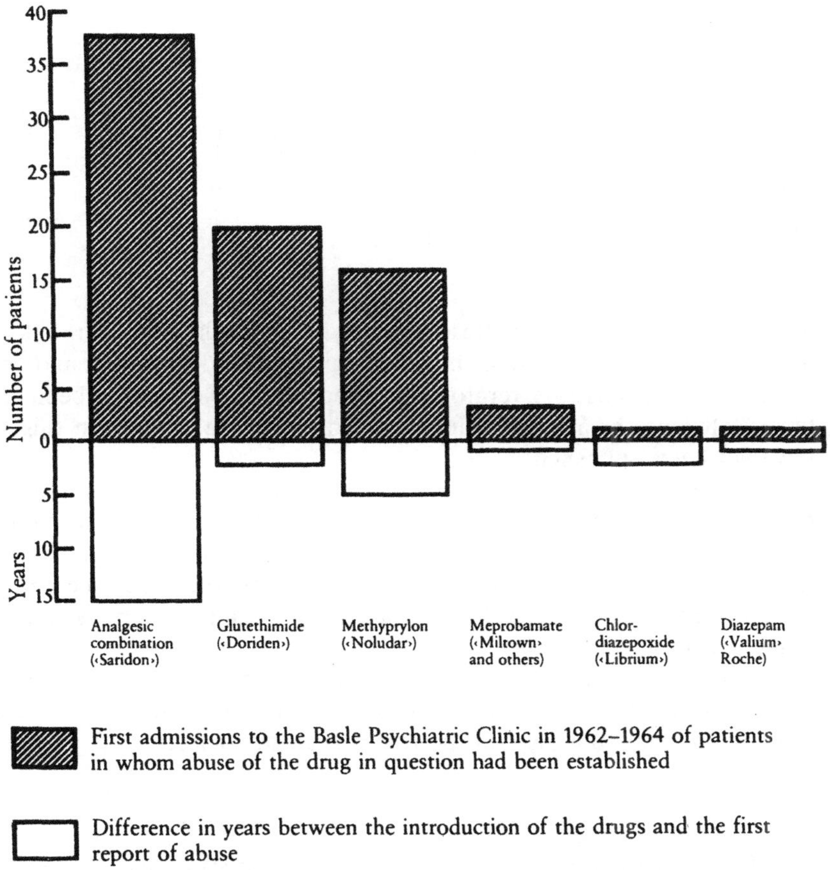

Fig. 16. Relationship between admission for drug abuse and the time span between the introduction of a drug and its abuse

tachyphylaxis they produce, can lead not only to addiction in the narrow sense but are also becoming an increasing object of abuse. With regard to the suicidal impulse, the danger consists mainly in the provocation of severe anxiety states. Keeler and Ungerleider (quoted by Ringel 1969b) and others have described suicide attempts under the influence of LSD. Another danger of the abuse of LSD or related substances is that chronic abuse can lead to severe personality changes. In susceptible individuals, acute psychoses may also be activated. So far experts differ in their assessments of the risk that LSD users will go on to truly addictive drugs such as heroin and cocaine. The same applies to marihuana or hashish, which is subject to increasing abuse, especially by young people. The crime syndicates are doubtless endeavouring to obtain new 'customers' in this way. Various investigations in the USA, particularly in the sociological field, have shown,

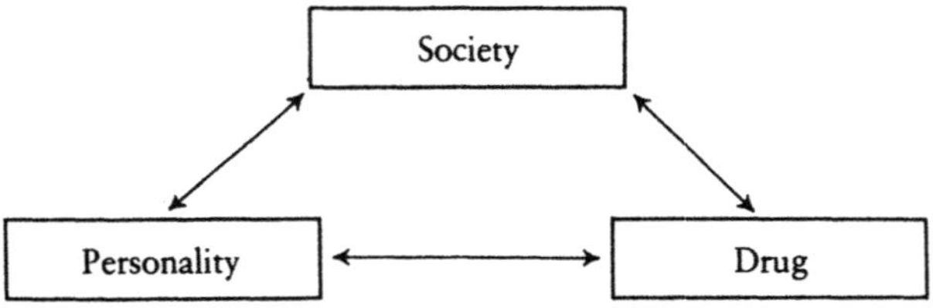

Fig. 17. Factors responsible for drug abuse

however, that people who abuse psycholytics, including hashish, belong to a different social stratum from those who are addicted to heroin and cocaine.

Recently a possible teratogenic effect of LSD has also been mooted (e.g. Zellweger et al.). No wide-scale and accurate studies on this subject have yet been published.

However, we must stress once again that phenomena of drug abuse and drug dependence can only be correctly assessed if one takes account of the interplay of drug, personality and society, as shown in Fig. 17. For the significance of the current attitude of society – its tolerance, encouragement or disapproval – is particularly clear in our main sociomedical problem, namely alcoholism.

Thus the borderline between the use and abuse of psychopharmaceuticals depends not only on their spectra of action and the personality structures of potential addicts, but also on the role played by society.

12.10 Psychotherapy and Psychopharmacotherapy

Before comparing and contrasting two different methods of treatment it should be realized that each may have entirely different points of departure and that it is not always possible to view them from the same angle. In order to illustrate this, let us consider the various approaches and theories that are of particular relevance to psychosomatics.

If one adopts what might be termed a psychobiological approach, the treatment arrived at is either psychopharmacotherapy or one of the various body therapies such as autogenic training. Should psychosomatic phenomena be regarded in a biographical light, i.e. a psychological approach be adopted, the method of treatment inevitably coming to mind is that known as client-centred psychotherapy, in which details of the life history are so important. If psychosomatic disorders and disease are viewed from a psychodynamic or depth-psychological angle, the trend is to analytic techniques. Again, one can regard the development of these illnesses from the aspect of learning theory, and then we have behaviour therapy and related methods of treatment. Finally, one can also see them from the angle of what meaning life has for the individual and we arrive at philosophically orientated solutions such as logotherapy and Dasein analysis.

In contrasting psychotherapy with psychopharmacotherapy we must accordingly not lose sight of the fact that two different points of departure are involved, namely the psychological (or depth-psychological) and the psychobiological. It must be emphasized that this is merely a matter of different ways of looking at things and not one of opposing principles; the different treatments developed from these aproaches by no means preclude one another. Let us consider for a moment the complex psychodynamics behind repressive and learning processes. These can take place only in the presence of functionally intact ganglion cells, which are indispensable for every psychological and psychosomatic event. This means one cannot simply cast aside the psychobiological approach. Indeed, it is a prime condition for the others.

Unfortunately however, the situation is such that the various schools of psychiatry, and especially psychotherapy, do not view the matter from the aspect of different approaches to the same end but rather from that of conflicting principles. This is not exactly a medical way of thinking; the purpose of diagnosis and treatment is not to confirm pet theories and accepted dogma. On the contrary, all members of the medical profession should feel themselves free to look to fresh strategies of treatment when those available fail, and even develop new ones. Despite this situation we do nevertheless have many different forms of treatment to fall back upon, ranging from client-centred therapy, analytic psychotherapy and behaviour therapy to philosophically orientated treatment such as logotherapy and Dasein analysis.

The problems involved in psychopharmacotherapy itself are somewhat less complex since we know what cerebral substrates individual drugs act upon and what general effects they produce. The main groups of psychotropic drugs at present available are neuroleptics, tranquilizers and antidepressants, which can be employed effectively in both mental and psychosomatic illness. It must, however, be realized that their effect is symptomatic and that they exert no direct influence on either extrapsychic or intrapsychic conflicts and problems. We thus return to the apparent antithesis of psychotherapy and psychopharmacotherapy. From today's standpoint we no longer see any truly opposing approaches since we can employ both psychotherapy and psychopharmacotherapy jointly. Although psychopharmaceuticals cannot solve the conflicts and problems just mentioned, the latter cannot in many cases be discussed with the patient in a meaningful manner until either the anxiolytic, tranquilizing or mood-elevating property of the drug has begun to take effect.

This is particularly true of psychosomatic disorders and diseases; the patient must be afforded some relief from his symptoms before embarking on what might prove to be a long course of psychotherapy. In this context

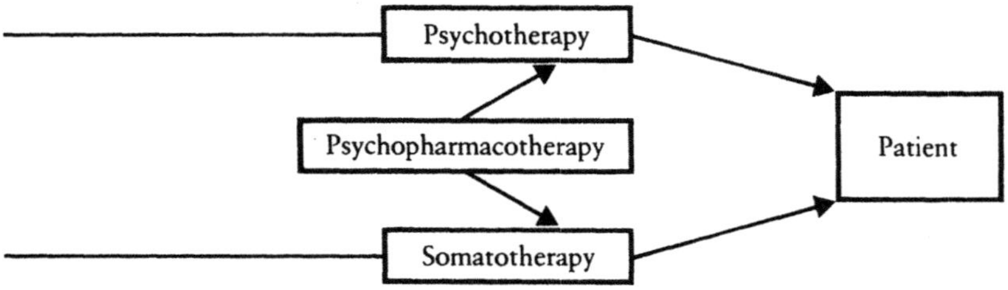

Fig. 18. Psychosomatically orientated plan of treatment

we should mention in particular the effect of the benzodiazepines on psycho-autonomic syndromes of restoring emotional equilibrium and dispelling anxiety.

While discussing the combination of these two mainstreams of treatment, it would be well to remember that in addition to the pharmacokinetic action of a drug there is also the effect produced by the doctor himself in prescribing it. The 'drug doctor', as Balint (1957a) described it, can play an important role in its efficacy. It is now widely known that the placebo effect is relatively high in psychotropic drugs, and that much depends upon both the manner in which a medicament is prescribed and the words used by the doctor at the time. While prescribing or administering such drugs we are to a certain extent not only in a position to exert a psychotherapeutic effect but also a somatotherapeutic action since some of them influence psycho-autonomic symptoms. These interrelationships between psychopharmacotherapy and psychotherapy on the one hand and somatotherapy on the other are summarized in Fig. 18. On giving this matter closer scrutiny we see that there is no conflict between psychopharmacotherapy and psychotherapy but rather that they are interlinked and can in turn influence purely somatotherapeutic aspects. Treatment with a psychotropic agent can bring about a condition under which the patient is more responsive to psychotherapy. Conversely, psychotherapy can promote the patient's understanding for the need to continue taking a drug for a prescribed period. A psychotropic drug can, moreover, have positive somatic effects and thus be of benefit to the patient's general well-being.

But how did the polarization of psychopharmacotherapy and psychotherapy come about? Historically speaking, psychiatry has always had its psychicists and somatists. The contrast between these two methods, of which such an issue has been made, is merely an interesting case of history repeating itself. Yet there is perhaps a practical issue we should mention. Only medical doctors (and dental surgeons in some countries) may prescribe and administer psychotropic agents, although we are fully aware that some non-medical people, particularly psychologists, can carry out excellent psychotherapy. From a 'politically professional' standpoint it is only to be expected that more opposition to psychotropic drugs thus stems from the echelons of the nonmedical psychotherapists than from those of the medical profession.

Summing up, we may say that a conflict along theoretical lines with historical backing could be construed between psychopharmacotherapy and psychotherapy. The clouds of conflict begin to disperse, however, as soon as it becomes evident we are not dealing with totally opposing principles but merely with different approaches. The doctor who does not set out with the idea of seeing pedantic notions and theories confirmed on each and every patient will inevitably seek out a wide range of therapeutic strategies in tune with his patient's individual needs. The most important and complementary forms of treatment for both psychic and psychosomatic disorders are psychotherapy and drug therapy. Where indicated they should of course be supplemented not only by somatotherapy but also by physiotherapy, ergotherapy, art therapy and music therapy. The wider the choice presented, the greater are the chances of success in treating each individual patient. Within this multifarious palette of possibilities, the psychotropic drug continues to occupy a prominent place.

13 References

Achté KB, Vankhonen ML (1970) Psychic factors in cancer. Cancer and psyche, p 1. Psychiatric Clinic of the University Central Hospital, Helsinki
Ackermann NW (ed) (1970) Family therapy in transition. Little Brown, Boston
Adler A (1920) Praxis und Theorie der Individualpsychologie. Bergmann, München
Aeschbacher A, Brunner T (1978) Die abnehmbare Teilprothese – eine Literaturübersicht. Schweiz Monatsschr Zahnheilkd 88:234
Ajuriaguerra J de (1966) Le médecin et la maladie. Présences 93:3
Alexander F (1934) Psychological factors in gastro-intestinal disturbances. Psychoanal Q 3:506
Alexander F (1939) Emotional factors in essential hypertension. Psychosom Med 1:175
Alexander F (1948) Fundamentals of psychoanalysis. Norton, New York
Alexander F (1950) Psychosomatic medicine, its principles and applications. Norton, New York
Alexander F (1951) Psychosomatische Medizin. De Gruyter, Berlin
Alexander F, French MT, Poolock GH (1968) Psychosomatic specifity. Experimental study and results. Univ Chicago Press, Chicago London
Argelander H (1963/64) Die Analyse psychischer Prozesse in der Gruppe. Psyche (Stuttg) 17:450
Argelander H (1966) Möglichkeiten der psychoanalytisch orientierten Psychotherapie in der ärztlichen Praxis. Saarl Ärztebl 6
Assal G (1976) La neuropsychologie peut-elle intéresser l'orthodontiste? Schweiz Monatsschr Zahnheilkd 86:342
Auden WH (1958) Das Zeitalter der Angst. Piper, München
Bach H (1969) Die Ausreifung der menschlichen Aggressivität (Am klinischen Beispiel der Tetanie und Schizphrenie). Fortsch Psychoanal 3:147
Baer PE (1983) Conflict management in the family. The impact of paternal hypertension. In: Advances in family intervention, assessment and theory, vol 3. JAI, Greenwich London
Baer PE, Vincent JP, Williams BJ, Bourianoff GG, Bartlett PC (1980) Behavioral response to induced conflict in families with a hypertensive father. Hypertension 2, I:70–77
Baer PE, Reed J, Bartlett PC, Vincent JP, Williams BJ, Bourianoff GG (1983) Studies of gaze during induced conflicts in families with a hypertensive father. Psychosom Med 45, 3:233–242
Bahnson CB (1967) Psychiatrisch-psychologische Aspekte bei Krebskranken. Verh Dtsch Ges Inn Med 73:536
Balabanski L, Tashev T (1976) The importance or regular psychological care of treated obese patients for maintainance of the reduced body weight. (Vortrag, Symposium: Diätische, psychologische und soziale Aspekte des Übergewichtes, Zürich 8.–9.9. 1976)
Balint M (1955) Psychotherapeutische Ausbildung des praktischen Arztes. Psyche (Stuttg) 9:370–389
Balint M (1957a) Der Arzt, sein Patient und die Krankheit. Klett, Stuttgart
Balint M (1957b) The doctor, his patient and the illness. Pitman, London

Balint M (1965) Die Urformen der Liebe und die Technik der Psychoanalyse. Klett, Stuttgart
Balint M (1968) Erfahrungen mit Ausbildungs- und Forschungsseminaren. Psyche (Stuttg)22:9–11
Balint M (1969) Die Urformen der Liebe und die Technik der Psychoanalyse. Fischer, Frankfurt
Baltrusch HJF (1969) Psychosomatische Beziehungen bei Krebskranken. Psychosom Med 7:196–219
Baltrusch HJF, Austerheim K, Baltrusch E (1963, 1964a,b) Psyche – Nervensystem – Neoplastischer Prozeβ: ein altes Problem mit neuer Aktualität. Z Psychosom Med 9:229, 10:1, 10:157
Barolin GS (1969) Migräne. Das angiozephale Attackensyndrom: Diagnostik, Ätiologie und Therapie. Facultas, Wien
Battegay R (1963) Angst als Ausdruck psychischen Krankseins. Schweiz Med Wochenschr 93:777
Battegay R (1966) Angst und ihre Beziehung zur Gruppe. Psychiatr Seelsorge 6
Battegay R (1967–1969) Der Mensch in der Gruppe, vols 1–3. Huber, Bern Stuttgart Wien
Battegay R (1970) Die psychosomatische Krankheit als Phänomen der Gruppe. (Vortrag, Jahresversammlung der Schweizerischen Gesellschaft für Psychosomatische Medizin, 22.–24.5. 1970)
Baumann M (1979) Atypische Gesichtsschmerzen. Schweiz Monatsschr Zahnheilkd 89:105
Beck D (1968) Die Kurzpsychotherapie. Schweiz Med Wochenschr 98:1859
Beck D (1969) Psychotherapie bei psychosomatischen Krankheiten. Habilitationsvortrag, Basel
Beck D (1971) Psychosomatische Aspekte des Weichteilrheumatismus. In: Forbildungskurse für Rheumatologie, vol 1. Karger, Basel, pp 168–177
Benedek T (1948) An approach to the study of the diabetic. Psychosom Med 10: 284–292
Bergdolt H, Ebschner K-J, Groβe-Ruyken F-J, Maiwald D, Nüssel E, Rotzler A, Schettler G (1986) Resümee von 15 Jahren epidemiologischer Herzinfarktforschung. Perspektiven für die Tätigkeit der niedergelassenen Ärzte. Dtsch Ärztebl 83, 10:607–613
Bergmann G von (1936) Funktionelle Pathologie. Springer, Berlin
Bergmann G (ed) (1989) Psychosomatische Grundversorgung. Springer, Berlin Heidelberg New York Tokyo
Bergmann G, Hahn P (1987) Die Bedeutung des sympathicovasalen Anfalles für die Nosologie und Therapie der herzphobischen Form der Herzneurose. In: Nutzinger D, Pfersmann D, Welan T, Zapotoczky HG (ed) Herzphobie. Enke, Stuttgart
Bergmann G, Kröger F, Petzold E (1986) Allgemeine klinische Psychosomatik – Weiterentwicklung eines Stationsmodells. Gruppenpsych Gruppendyn 21:224–235
Bernheim E (1978) Contribution à l'étude des relations entre l'humour et l'art dentaire. Dissertation, Straβburg University
Bernsheimer A (1967) Häufigkeit und Ursachen der verschiedenen Hochdruckformen. Münch Med Wochenschr 109:1837
Bertalanffy L von (1973) General systems theory. Pinguin, Harmondsworth
Berufsbild „Zahnarzt 2000" der Schweizerischen Zahnärzte-Gesellschaft (1986) pp 31–36
Billeter A (1978) Problem der Arzt-Patienten-Beziehung beim Tumorkranken. (Vortrag, 1. Ostschweizerische Ärzte-Fortbildungstage „Onkologie und Hämatologie für die Praxis")
Binder H (1949) Über die Angst. Schweiz Med Wochenschr 79:705–711
Binswanger L (1955) Ausgewählte Vorträge und Aufsätze. Francke, Bern

Binswanger L (1957) Schizophrenie (Kap. „Der Fall Ellen West"). Neske, Pfullingen
Birkmayer W (1970) Der Verlust der humanen Integration. Monatsh Ärztl Fortbild 20:54
Bleuler E (1975) Lehrbuch der Psychiatrie, 13th edn. Springer, Berlin Heidelberg New York
Bleuler M (1961) Entwicklungslinien psychiatrischer Praxis und Forschung in jüngster Zeit. Schweiz Med Wochenschr 91:1549
Bleuler M (1970) Bleiben wir am Kranken. Schweiz Ärzteztg 51:203–232
Blohmke M (1976) Psychosoziale Faktoren und Krankheit. Med Mensch Ges 1:116–121
Blomfield LB (1964) Rheumatism and emotion. In: Hoff H, Tschabitscher H, Kryspin-Exner K (eds) Muskel und Psyche. Karger, Basel New York, S 142–149
Boss M (1954) Einführung in die psychosomatische Medizin. In: Rossier PH, Spühler O (eds) Innere Medizin und ihre Grenzgebiete, Bd 6. Huber, Bern Stuttgart Wien
Boszormenyi-Nagy I, Sparke M (1981) Unsichtbare Bindungen. Klett-Cotta, Stuttgart
Bräutigam W (1969) Reaktionen – Neurosen – Psychopathien. Thieme, Stuttgart
Bräutigam W (1976) Psychosomatische Gesichtspunkte zu Genese und Therapie der Übergewichtigkeit. Therapiewoche 26:1206–1212
Bräutigam W, Christian P (1973) Psychosomatische Medizin. Thieme, Stuttgart
Brecht B (1976) Die unwürdige Greisin. Gesammelte Werke 11. Suhrkamp, Frankfurt am Main, pp 315–320
Bregulla-Beyer S (1988) Der Aufbau von Anamnesegruppen in Heidelberg 1979–1982: Ein Beispiel studentischer Eigeninitiative in der Ausbildung zum Arzt. In: Schüffel W (ed) Sich gesund fühlen im Jahre 2000. Springer, Berlin Heidelberg New York Tokyo
Bronkhorst W (1950) Das psychische Moment bei der Behandlung der Lungentuberkulose. Psyche (Stuttg) 3:721
Bruch H (1957) The importance of overweight. Norton, New York
Bruch H (1971) Death in anorexia nervosa. Psychosom Med 33:135–144
Bruch H (1973) Eating disorders. Basic Books, New York
Bruch H (1980) Der goldene Käfig. Das Rätsel der Magersucht. Fischer, Frankfurt am Main
Busch W (o.J.) Gesamtausgabe. Vollmer, Wiesbaden
Buser M (1971) Die Chronizität in ihrer psychosomatischen Bedingtheit. Bibl Tuberc Med Thora 27:44–56
Calanca A (1988) Vade-mecum de thérapeutique psychiatrique, 6th edn. Bettex, Lausanne Paris
Cannon WB (1975) Wut, Hunger, Angst und Schmerz, Urban & Schwarzenberg, München Berlin Wien
Cathomen-Rötheli M, Hobi V, Graber G (1976) Untersuchungen über die Persönlichkeitsstruktur an Myoarthropathie erkrankten Patienten. Schweiz Monatsschr Zahnheilkd 86:29
Christian P (1975) Grundlagen der Psychosomatik. Z Klin Psychol Psychother 23:303–308
Christian P, Mohr P, Ulmer W (1955) Das nervöse Atmungssyndrom bei Vegetativ-Labilen. Dtsch Arch Inn Med 201:702
Christian P, Fink-Eikel K, Huber W (1966) Risikofaktoren und Risikopersönlichkeit beim Herzinfarkt. Verh Dtsch Ges Kreislaufforsch 32:97
Clauser G (1967) Psychotherapie-Fibel. Thieme, Stuttgart
Clemmesen C (1963) Die Kopenhagener Methode zur Behandlung narkotischer Vergiftungen. Med Welt 3:1095
Cobb S (1959) Contained hostility in rheumatoid arthritis. Arthritits Rheum 2:419
Cobb S (1962) Hostility and its control in rheumatoid disease. Arthritis Rheum 5:290
Condrau G (1965) Psychosomatik der Frauenheilkunde. Huber, Bern Stuttgart Wien

Condrau G (1969) Bedeutung der medizinischen Psychologie für die ärztliche Praxis. Psychosom Med 4:111
Cooper B (1964) The epidemiological approach to psychosomatic medicine. J Psychosom Res 8:9
Cooper JC (1977) Tooth exfoliation and osteonecrosis of the jaw following Herpes Zoster. Br Dent J 143:297
Cremerius J (1965) Zur Prognose der Anorexia nervosa. Arch Psychiatr Z Ges Neurol 207:378–393
Cremerius J (1968) Die Prognose funktioneller Syndrome. Enke, Stuttgart
De Beauvoir S (1968) Das andere Geschlecht. Rowohlt, Reinbek bei Hamburg
De Boor C (1959) Über den Widerstand gegen die psychosomatische Therapie. Ärztl Prax11:46
De Boor C (1965) Zur Psychosomatik der Allergie, insbesondere des Asthma bronchiale, vol 4. Huber & Klett, Bern Stuttgart Wien
De Boor C, Künzler E (1963) Die psychosomatische Klinik und ihre Patienten. Huber/Klett, Bern Stuttgart
Delius L (1975) Modelle sozialer Einwirkungen auf den Menschen. Psychosomatische Konzepte. In: Blohmke M, Ferber C, Kisker KP, Schäfer H (eds) Handbuch der Sozialmedizin, vol 1. Enke, Stuttgart, p 133
Delius L, Fahrenberg J (1986) Psychovegetative Syndrome. Thieme, Stuttgart
Deter HC (1986) Psychosomatische Behandlung des Asthma bronchiale: Indikation, Therapie und Ergebnisse der krankheitszentrierten Gruppentherapie. Springer, Berlin Heidelberg New York Tokyo
Deter HC, Petzold E, Hengst-Theis R, Breiden U, Lanzinger-Rossnagel G (1983) Katamnestische Ergebnisse einer klinisch-psychosomatischen Behandlung von 103 Patienten mit Anorexia nervosa aus internistischer Sicht. Innere Med 10:3–12
Deutsch F (1939) Associative anamnesis. Psychoanal Q 8:354
Deutsch F (1953) The psychosomatic concept in psychoanalysis. Int Univ Press, New York
Deutsch F (1964) Training in psychosomatic medicine. Hafner, New York
Deyhle P, Jenny S (1976) Ulcus duodeni. Endoskopiebefund und psychosozialer Status. Department für Innere Medizin der Universität Zürich, Zürich
DSM-III-R (1989) Diagnostisches und statistisches Manual psychischer Störungen. Deutsche Bearbeitung und Einführung von Wittchen HU, Saβ H, Zauding M, Koehler K. Beltz, Weinheim Basel
Dolder E (1956) Zur Psychologie des Zahnverlustes und des Zahnersatzes. Dtsch Zahnärztl Z 11:469
Drommer R (1979) Das Zervikalsyndrom. Schweiz Monatsschr Zahnheilkd 89:520
Dunbar F (1947) Mind and body: Psychosomatic medicine. Random, New York
Dunbar F (1948) Psychosomatic diagnosis. Hoeber, New York
Dunbar F (1954) Emotions and bodily changes, 4th edn. Columbia Univ Press, New York
Duss-von Werth J, Hauser GA (1970) Das Buch von Liebe und Ehe. Walter, Olten Freiburg
Edwards G (1969) The british approach to the treatment of heroin addiction. Lancet I:768–772
Ehrenfels C von (1890) Über Gestaltqualitäten. Vjwiss Phil 14:249–292
Eichhorn O (1950/51) Daseinsanalytische Anmerkungen zu den zentralbedingten vegetativen Regulationsstörungen. Psyche (Heidelberg) 4:352–357
Elhardt S (1962) Über den Umgang mit schwierigen Patienten. Dtsch Zahnärztl Z 17:1253
Engel GL (1967) The concept of psychosomatic disorder. J Psychosom Res 11:3
Engel GL (1970) Psychisches Verhalten in Gesundheit und Krankheit (Translation Adler R). Huber, Bern Stuttgart Wien
Engel GL, Schmale A Jr (1976) Psychoanalytic theory of somatic disorder:

Conversion, specificity, and the disease onset stituation. J Am Psychoanal Assoc 15:344
Engel GL, Schmale AH (1968) A life-setting conducive to illness: The giving-up, given-up complex. Am Intern Med 69:293–300
Engel GL, Schmale A Jr (1969) Eine psychoanalytische Theorie der somatischen Störung. Psyche (Stuttg) 23:241
English OS (1952) Médicine psychosomatique. Delachaux & Niestlé, Neuenburg Paris
Fain M (1966) Régression et psychosomatique. Rev Fr Psychoanal 30:451
Farrelly F, Brandsma J (1986) Provokative Therapie. Springer, Berlin Heidelberg New York Tokyo
Ferenczi S (1965) Bausteine zur Psychoanalyse. Huber, Bern Stuttgart Wien
Fox BH, Stanekey G, Boyd SC (1983) Suicide rates among cancer patients in Connecticut. Manuscript National Cancer Institute, Bethesda
Framo JL (ed) (1972) Family interaction. Springer, Berlin Heidelberg New York
Framo JL (1975) Beweggründe und Techniken der intensiven Familientherapie. In: Boszormenyi-Nagy I, Framo JL (eds) Familientherapie. Therapie und Praxis, vol 2. Rowohlt, Reinbek bei Hamburg
Frankl VE (1947) Die Psychotherapie in der Praxis. Deuticke, Wien
Frankl VE (1975) Theorie und Therapie der Neurosen. UTB, Reinhardt, München
Freud S (published 1961a) Über die Berechtigung von der Neurasthenie einen bestimmten Symptomkomplex als „Angstneurose" abzutrennen. Gesammelte Werke vol 1, Fischer, Frankfurt
Freud S (published 1961b) Vorlesungen zur Einführung in die Psychoanalyse. Gesammelte Werke vol 9. Fischer, Frankfurt
Freyberger H (1969) Psychosomatische Therapie bei Colitis Ulcerosa. Med Klin 64:969
Freyberger H (1972) Der psychosomatische Umgang mit Patienten mit Magen- und Zwölffingerdarmgeschwür. Therapiewoche 23:2492
Freyberger H (1976a) Psychosoziale Probleme bei Herzinfarktpatienten. Therapiewoche 26:5510–5514
Freyberger H (1976b) „Symptom", „Konflikt" und „Persönlichkeit" in der Behandlung psychosomatischer Patienten. Prax Psychother 3:121–131
Freyberger H, Leutner V (1974) Die psychosomatische Therapie des Magen- und Zwölffingerdarmgeschwürs. Therapiewoche 24:278
Freyberger H, Struwe H (1962/63) Psychosomatische Aspekte der Fettsucht. Psyche (Stuttg) 16:561
Fromm E (1964) Psychoanalyse und Ethik, 2nd edn. Diana, Konstanz Zürich
Fromm E (1966) Psychoanalyse und Religion. Diana, Konstanz Zürich
Fromm E (1968) Das Menschliche in uns. Diana, Konstanz Zürich
Fromm-Reichmann F (1959) Intensive Psychotherapie. Hippokrates, Stuttgart
Fuchs M (1965) Der Weiberschlapp. Verlauf einer Asthmaheilung. Prax Kinderpsychol 6:209–213
Gastpar M (1985) Relevante Forschungsergebnisse für die Praxis. Inf Arzt 2a:8–12
Gastpar M (1986) Möglichkeiten und Grenzen der Depressionsbehandlung in der Praxis. Ther Umschau 43:5055
Gaupp R (1910) Über den Selbstmord. München
Gebsattel VE von (1954) Prolegomena einer medizinischen Anthropologie. Springer, Berlin Göttingen Heidelberg
Gentz A (1983) Führung und Behandlung ängstlicher und behinderter Kinder. Schweiz Monatsschr Zahnheilkd 93:861–865
Gerlach D, Wolters H (1977) Zahn- und Mundschleimhautbefunde bei Rauschmittelkonsumenten. Dtsch Zahnärztl Z 32:400
Giesecke N, Luban-Plozza B, Rappel-Giesecke K (eds) (1983) Kommunikation in Balintgruppen. Patientenbezogene Medizin 6. Fischer, Stuttgart New York

Glatzel H (1954) Zur Psychosomatik der Ulcuskrankheit: Ergebnisse einer klinischen Arbeitsrichtung. Z Psychosom Med 1:11–21
Goldschmidt O (1973) Die funktionelle Sterilität der Frau. Psyche (Stuttg) 27:69–86
Greco RS, Pittenger RA (1968) Ein Hausarzt und seine Praxis. Klett, Stuttgart
Groddeck G (1961a) Das Buch vom Es. Limes, Wiesbaden
Groddeck G (1961b) Psychoanalytische Schriften zur Psychosomatik. Limes, Wiesbaden
Groen JJ, Loos WS de (1973) Psychosomatische aspecten van diabetes mellitus. Amsterdam
Groos F (1824) Über etwas nicht Mönchisches, sondern Sokratisches, was der Heilkunst Noth thut. Z Anthropol
Grossarth-Maticek R (1976) Krebserkrankung und Familie. Z Familienther 4:294–318
Grossarth-Maticek R (1978) Wer sich exponiert ist gefährdet. Psychol Heute 6:32–39
Grossarth-Maticek R (1979) Krankheit als Biographie. Kiepenheuer & Witsch, Köln
Grubbe P (o.J.) Verschenkte Jahre. Praeger, München Wien Zürich
Gunthern G (1982) Auto-Organisation in Humansystemen. In: Zusammenhänge 3, Menschliche Systeme: Ein Rahmen für das Denken, die Forschung und das Handeln. Institut für Ehe und Familie, Zürich
Gunthern G (1984) Systemtherapie und die sogenannte psychosomatische Frage. Kassenarzt 24:40 ff
Gutter A, Luban-Plozza B (1978) Familie als Risiko und Chance. Antonius, Solothurn
Habermas T, Müller M (1986) Das Bulimiesyndrom: Krankheitsbild, Dynamik und Therapie. Nervenarzt 57:322–331
Haefely W (1980) Wie wirken Benzodiazepine? Neuestes aus der Psychopharmakaforschung. (Habilitationsvorlesung, unpublished)
Hahn P (1965) Zur Analyse der auslösenden Situation bei der sogenannten „Herzphobie“. Z Psychosom Med 11:264–280
Hahn P (1969) Über die Indikation zu verschiedenen psychotherapeutischen Verfahren. Hippokrates 40:941–950
Hahn P (1971) Der Herzinfarkt in psychosomatischer Sicht. Vandenhoeck & Ruprecht, Göttingen
Hahn P (ed) (1979) Psychologie des 20. Jahrhunderts, vol IX. Ergebnisse für die Medizin (1). Psychosomatische Medizin. Kindler, Zürich
Hahn P (1988) Ärztliche Propädeutik – Gespräch, Anamnese Interview. Springer, Berlin Heidelberg New York Tokyo
Hahn P, Nüssel E, Stieler M (1966) Psychosomatik und Epidemiologie des Herzinfarktes. Z Psychosom Med 12:229–253
Hahn P, Mayer H, Stanek W (1973) Biometrische Befunde bei der Herzneurose. Z Psychosom Med Psychoanal 19:231–264
Haley J (1977) Direktive Familientherapie. Strategien für die Lösung von Problemen. Pfeiffer, München
Haley J (1978) Gemeinsamer Nenner Interaktion. Strategien der Psychotherapie. Pfeiffer, München
Heidegger M (1963) Sein und Zeit. Niemeyer, Tübingen
Heim E (1966a) Grenzen und Möglichkeiten der psychosomatischen Medizin. 1. Theoretische und experimentelle Aspekte. Schweiz Med Wochenschr 96:1717–1722
Heim E (1966b) Grenzen und Möglichkeiten der psychosomatischen Medizin. II. Klinische Aspekte. Schweiz Med Wochenschr 96:1751–1755
Heim E, Blaser A, Waidelich E (1970) Dyspnoe: Eine psychosomatische Untersuchung. Respiration 27:1–23
Heinroth JC (1818) Lehrbuch der Störungen des Seelenlebens oder der Seelenstörungen und ihrer Behandlung. Vogel, Leibzig

Herzog W, Petzold E, Kröger F (1988) Die Elterngruppe als flankierende Maßnahme bei der Behandlung von Anorexia nervosa-Patienten. In: Deter HC (ed) Gruppen mit körperlich Kranken. Eine Therapie auf verschiedenen Ebenen. Springer, Berlin Heidelberg New York Tokyo
Hinkle LE Jr (1961) Ecological observations of the relation of physical illness, mental illness, and the social environment. Psychosom Med 23:289
Hinkle LE Jr (1964) Human ecology, 'psychosomatic medicine' and the medical curriculum. Adv Psychosom Med 4:23
Hoff H, Ringel E (1964) Aktuelle Probleme der psychosomatischen Medizin. Jolis, München
Holz J (1978) Principes d'une réhabilitation orale raisonnable. Schweiz Monatsschr Zahnheilkd 88:935
Huebschmann H (1952) Psyche und Tuberkulose. Enke, Stuttgart (Beiträge aus der allgemeinen Medizin, vol 8)
Jackson DD (1980) Der Mythos der Normalität. In: Watzlawick P, Weakland JH (eds) Interaktion. Huber, Bern
Jacobi J (1965) Der Weg zur Individuation. Rascher, Zürich Stuttgart
Jacobson E (1938) Progressive relaxation. Univ Chicago Press, Chicago
Jaspers K (1965) Allgemeine Psychopathologie, 8th edn. Springer, Berlin Heidelberg New York
Jenkins CD (1972) Psychologic and social precursors of coronary disease. N Engl J Med 284:244
Johnson L, Flach A (1985) Family characteristics of 105 Patients with bulimia. Am J Psychiatry 142:1321–1324
Jores A (1970) Der Mensch und seine Krankheit. Huber & Klett, Bern Stuttgart Wien
Jores A (1976) Praktische Psychosomatik. Huber, Bern Stuttgart Wien
Joris R (1977) Aspects juridiques et cliniques des échecs en médicine dentaire. Schweiz Monatsschr Zahnheilkd 87:842
Jung CG (1950) Seelenprobleme der Gegenwart, 5th edn. Rascher, Zürich Stuttgart
Junge B (1988) Sterblichkeit im mittleren Lebensalter. Neue Ärztliche 54:11
Junker H (1972) Ehepaargruppentherapie mit Patienten aus der oberen Unterschicht. Psyche (Stuttg) 26:541–556
Karush A, Danils G, O'Connor JF, Stern LO (1968) The response to psychotherapy in chronic ulcerative colitis. Psychosom Med 3:255–262
Kast V (1982) Trauern. Kreuz, Stuttgart
Kempler W (1975) Grundzüge der Gestalt-Familientherapie. Klett-Cotta, Stuttgart
Kielholz P (ed) (1966) Angst – psychische und somatische Aspekte. Huber, Bern Stuttgart Wien
Kielholz P (1967) Vergleichende Untersuchungen über Genese und Verlauf der Drogenabhängigkeit und des Alkoholismus. Schweiz Med Wochenschr 97:893–944
Kielholz P (1968) Gesamtschweizerische Enquête über die Häufigkeit des Medikamentenmißbrauches. Schweiz Ärzteztg 40:1077
Kielholz P (1971) Diagnose und Therapie der Depressionen für den Praktiker, 3rd edn. Lehmann, München
Kielholz P (ed) (1973) Die larvierte Depression. Huber, Bern Stuttgart Zürich
Kielholz P (1974) Psychopharmaka in der Zahnheikunde und Drogenabhängigkeit. Schweiz Monatsschr Zahnheilkd 84:1007
Kielholz P (ed) (1981) Der Allgemeinpraktiker und seine depressiven Patienten. Huber, Bern Stuttgart Wien
Kielholz P (ed) (1982) Antidepressiva-Infusionstherapie. Thieme, Stuttgart
Kielholz P, Pöldinger W, Adams C (1981) Die larvierte Depression. Ein didaktisches Konzept zur Diagnose und Therapie somatisierter Depressionen. Deutscher Ärzte-Verlag, Köln
Kierkegaard S (1960) Der Begriff der Angst. Rowohl, Reinbek bei Hamburg

Kind H (1966) Möglichkeiten zur Ausbildung in Psychotherapie für den praktizierenden Arzt. Ther Umsch 23:267
Kissen D, Le Shan LL (eds) (1964) Psychosomatic aspects of neoplastic disease. Pitman, London
Kleinknecht RA (1976) Psychology and dentistry. Prof Psychol 7:4
Klußmann R (1986) Psychosomatische Medizin. Springer, Berlin Heidelberg New York Tokyo
Knoepfel HK (1961) Einfache Psychotherapie für den Hausarzt. Huber, Bern Stuttgart Wien
Knoepfel HK (1968/1969) Hausärztliche Psychotherapie auf analytischer Basis. Psychosom Med 1:2
Knoepfel HK (1970) Hausärztliche Psychotherapie und Arzt-Patienten-Beziehung. Praxis 59:314–319
Koch U, Schmeling C (1978) Umgang mit Sterbenden – ein Lernprogramm für Ärzte, Medizinstudenten und Krankenschwestern. Med Psychol 4:81–93
Köhle K, Simons C (1979) Anorexia nervosa. In: Uexküll T von (ed) Lehrbuch der psychosomatischen Medizin. Urban & Schwarzenberg, München Wien Baltimore, p 529
Körber E (1978) Die zahnärztliche prothetische Versorgung des älteren Menschen. Hanser, München Wien
Kranz H (1965) Gebrauch und Mißbrauch der Psychopharmaka in der allgemeinen Praxis. Ergebnis einer Umfrage. Ärztebl Rheinl-Pfalz 18:147
Krehl L von (1936) Krankheitsform und Persönlichkeit. Vogel, Leibzig
Kröger F, Luban-Plozza B (eds) (1982) Studenten-Balint-Gruppen (Junior-Balint-Gruppen). Eine Erweiterung der medizinischen Ausbildung. Patientenbezogene Medizin 4. Fischer, Stuttgart New York
Kröger F, Petzold E (1985) Klinische Psychosomatik: Blutdruckregulation. Problemstellung aus systemtheoretischer Sicht. Z Psychosom Med 31:339–354
Kröger F, Hahn P, Senges J (1985a) Funktionelle Herzbeschwerden. Klinik – Differentialdiagnose – Therapie. Dtsch Ärztebl 82, 27:2017–2021
Kröger F, Hahn P, Senges J (1985b) Funktionelle Herzbeschwerden. Spezielle Krankheitsbilder. Dtsch Ärztebl 82, 28/29:2116–2118
Kröger F, Bergmann G, Petzold E (1986) Klinische Psychosomatik: Individuelle Aufnahmesituation und systemisches Symptomverständnis. Ist ein Brückenschlag möglich? Z System Ther 4 (1):10–17
Krüskemper GM, Krüskemper HL (1976) Die Psychosomatik der Kranken mit Schilddrüsenleiden: In: Jores A (ed) Praktische Psychosomatik. Huber, Bern Stuttgart Wien, p 302
Kütemeyer W (1956) Anthropologische Medizin in der inneren Klinik. In: Arzt im Irrsal der Zeit. Vandenhoeck & Ruprecht, Göttingen
Kuhn R (1953) Zur Daseinsanalyse der Anorexia mentalis. 2. Studie. Nervenarzt 24:191
Kübler-Ross E (1974) Interviews mit Sterbenden. Kreuz, Berlin (Gütersloher Taschenbücher Bd 71)
Labhardt F (1965) Der seelische Zugang zum körperlich Kranken. Schweiz Ärzteztg 2:42–43
Labhardt F (1970) Vielfalt und Problematik vegetativer Funktion und Störungen. Psychosom Med 1:88–91
Lambert P, Revol L (1960) Classification psychopharmacologique et clinique des différents neuroleptiques. Presse Med 68:1509–1511
Leatherman G (1978) Zukünftige Verpflichtungen der Zahnheilkunde. Schweiz Monatsschr Zahnheilkd 5:217
Le Shan (1982) Psychotherapie gegen den Krebs. Klett-Cotta, Stuttgart
Lewis BI (1957) Hyperventilation syndroms: clinical and physiologic observations. Postgrad Med 21:259–271
Lichtwitz L (1936) Pathologie der Funktionen und Regulationen. Sijtnoff, Leiden

Loch W (1963) Regression. Psyche (Stuttg) 17:516
Loebell E (1976) Phoniatrie und ihre Beziehungen zur Kieferorthopädie. Schweiz Monatsschr Zahnheilkd 86:327
Loew D (1965) Suizidversuche mit Psychopharmaka im Patientengut einer psychiatrischen Universitätsklinik. Ther Umsch 22:186–188
Luban-Plozza B (1969) Aspects psychosomatiques de la médicine dentaire. Méd Hyg 27:1116–1118
Luban-Plozza B (ed) (1989) Der psychosomatische Zugang – Chance für Patient und Arzt. Perimed, Frankfurt am Main
Luban-Plozza B, Balint E (eds) (1978) Patientenbezogene Medizin. 1. Balint-Methode in der medizinischen Ausbildung. Fischer, Stuttgart New York
Luban-Plozza B, Dickhaut HD (eds) (1984) Praxis der Balint-Gruppen. Beziehungsdiagnostik und Therapie. Springer, Berlin Heidelberg New York
Luban-Plozza B, Loch W (eds) (1979) Psychotherapie in der Sprechstunde. Patientenbezogene Medizin 2. Fischer, Stuttgart New York
Luban-Plozza B, Meerloo JAM (1968) Anorexie mentale et suicide intestinal. Med Hyg 26:847
Luban-Plozza B, Knaak L, Dickhaut HD (1987) Der Arzt als Arzenei. Deutscher Ärzte-Verlag, Köln
Luban-Plozza B, Delli Ponti N, Dickhaut HD (1988) Musik und Psyche. Birkhäuser, Basel Boston
Maeder A (1953) La personne du médecin. Delachaux & Niestlé, Neuenburg Paris
Maeder A (1963) Studien über Kurzpsychotherapie. Klett, Stuttgart
Magri F (1983) Psychologie in der Prophylaxe bei Jugendlichen und Randgruppen. Schweiz Monatsschr Zahnheilkd 93:820–828
Manné J (1970) Psychologie et art dentaire: L'unit, L'ambiance, l'exercice logique. Ann Odonto-Stomatol 27:153
Marcel G (1955) Etre et avoir. Paris
Marthaler T (1978) Ist Zahnlosigkeit im Zurückgehen begriffen? Schweiz Monatsschr Zahnheilkd 88:1036
Marty P (1974) Die „allergische Objektbeziehung". In: Brede K (ed) Einführung in die psychosomatische Medizin. Athenäum Fischer, Frankfurt, p 420
Marty P, M'Uzan M de (1963) La pensée opératoire. Rev Fr Psychoanal [Suppl] 27:1345–1356
Masters WH, Johnson VE (1970) Die sexuelle Reaktion. Rowohlt, Reinbek bei Hamburg
Masters WH, Johnson VE (1973) Impotenz und Anorgasmie. Goverts Krüger Stahlberg, Frankfurt am Main
Matthes I (1974) Ein Urticaria-Patient. Versuch einer Darstellung seines Selbsterlebens anhand von Auszügen aus dem Rorschach-Test. In: Brede K (ed) Einführung in die Psychosomatische Medizin. Athenäum Fischer, Frankfurt am Main
Maudsley H (1876) The physiology of mind. Macmillan, London
May G, Squazorni AT (1969) Problémes psychologiques dans les traitements dentaires des enfants. Rev Mens Swisse Odonto-Stomatol 79:719
Mayer H (1975) Das Herz als Spiegel der Seele (Befund und Befinden). Z Klin Psychol Psychother 23:309–315
Meerloo JAM (1971) Difficultés d'adaptation dans le troisième âge. Praxis 60:32
Meerwein F (1960) Über die Führung des ersten Gesprächs. Schweiz Med Wochenschr 90:497
Meerwein F (1969) Die Grundlagen des ärztlichen Geprächs. Huber, Bern Stuttgart Wien
Meier O (1968) Psychotherapie in der Allgemeinpraxis. (Vorträge des 12. Internationalen IMA-Seminars, Mariazell, Kongreßhefte)
Mellgren A (1978) Zahnersatz und Psyche. Sexualmedizin 7:420–428
Meng H (1934) Das Problem der Organpsychose. Int Z Psychoanal 20:439

Meng H (1935) Organische Erkrankung als Organpsychose. Schweiz Arch Neurol Psychiatr 36:271
Meyer AE (1976) Die Psychosomatik der Ulkuskranken. In: Jores A (ed) Praktische Psychosomatik. Huber, Bern Stuttgart Wien, p 175
Minuchin S (1977) Familie und Familientherapie. Lambertus, Freiburg
Minuchin S, Rosman B, Baker L (1983) Psychosomatische Krankheiten in der Familie. Klett-Cotta, Stuttgart
Mirsky IA (1958) Physiologic, psychologic and social determants in the etiology of duodenal ulcer. Am J Dig Dis 3:285
Mitscherlich A (1956) Krankheit als Konflikt, vols 1–2. Suhrkamp, Frankfurt am Main
Mitscherlich A (1961/62) Anmerkungen über die Chronifizierung psychosomatischen Geschehens. Psyche (Stuttg) 15:1
Mitterauer B (1981) Das suizidale Achsensyndrom. Eine medizinisch biologische Studie zur Abschätzung der Suizidalität. Wien Med Wochenschr [Suppl] 68:1–29
Moser U (1964) Gesprächsführung und Interviewtechnik. Psychol Rundsch 15:263–282
Müller C (1967) Alterspsychiatrie. Thieme, Stuttgart
Müller W (1968) Psychotrope Pharmaka in der Rheumatologie. In: Kranksein in seiner organischen und psychischen Dimension. Hoffmann-La Roche, Grenzach, pp 209–221
Müller-Eckhard H (1970) Das unverstandene Kind. Klett, Stuttgart
Müller-Fahlbusch W (1977) Psychosomatische Gesichtspunkte zur Differentialdiagnose zwischen Protheseninsuffizienz und Prothesenunverträglichkeit. Schriftenreihe der Bezirksärztekammer Stuttgart, Stuttgart
Müller-Fahlbusch W (1983) Kritische Anmerkungen zur psychogenen Prothesenunverträglichkeit. Schweiz Monatsschr Zahnheilkd 93:882–890
Musaph H (1976) Die Psychosomatik dermatologisch Kranker. In: Jores A (ed) Praktische Psychosomatik. Huber, Bern Stuttgart Wien, S 344
Noelpp B, Noelpp-Eschenhagen J (1951) Das experimentelle Asthma bronchiale des Meerschweinchens. Int Arch Allergy 2:308–321
Nutzinger D, Pfersmann D, Welan T, Zapotoczky HG (eds) (1987) Herzphobie. Enke, Stuttgart
Oestereich K (1975) Psychiatrie des Alterns. Quelle & Mayer, Heidelberg
Overbeck G, Biebl W (1975) Psychosomatische Modellvorstellungen zur Pathogenese der Ulcuskrankheit. Psyche (Stuttg) 29:542
Pakesch E (1974) Die Familie als Patient. Akad Druck-Z und Verlagsanstalt, Graz
Parade GW (1970) Orthostasestörung und zentral wirkende Substanzen. Ärztl Praxis 22:4255
Pavlov IP (1927) Conditioned Reflexes. Trans. GV Anrep, London: Oxford University Press
Perko M (1979) Das Zungenbrennen. Schweiz Monatsschr Zahnheilkd 89:120
Petzold E (1976) Psychotherapeutische Gesichtspunkte bei der Nachbehandlung von Patienten mit Herzinfarkt. Notabene Medici 6:14–18
Petzold E (1978) Individuelle und familiendynamische Gesichtpunkte bei Herzinfarktpatienten. (Habilitationsvorlesung, Heidelberg, unpublished)
Retzold E (1979) Familienkonfrontationsherapie bei Anorexia nervosa. Verlag für Medizinische Psychologie im Verlag Vanenhoeck & Ruprecht, Göttingen Zürich
Petzold E (1983) Anorexia nervosa. In: Luban-Plozza B, Matern HJ, Wesiak W (eds) Der Zugang zum psychosomatischen Denken. Hilfe für den niedergelassenen Arzt. Springer, Berlin Heidelberg New York Tokyo
Petzold E (1984a) Über den systemischen Zugang in der Balintarbeit. Materialien zur Psychoanalyse X:252–267
Petzold E (ed) (1984b) Klinische Wege zur Balint-Arbeit. Die Zugänge zur Balint-Arbeit aus der inneren Medizin und Chirurgie. Fischer, Stuttgart
Petzold E (1988a) Der andere Weg zum Patienten. Gedanken zur Balint-Arbeit. Krankenhausarzt 61:7

Petzold E (1988b) Kontrolle, Reglementierung und Freiheit im Alter aus der Sicht eines Psychosomatikers. (Seniorenakademie Heidelberg, unpublished manuscript)
Petzold E, Bergmann G (1986) Konfrontation im Systemischen (KIS). Die Familiendimension in einem klinischen System. Prax Psychother Psychosom 31:87–95
Petzold E, Hahn P (1974) Zur Problematik des Syndromwandels. Prax Psychother 2:14
Petzold E, Reindell A (1977) Psychosomatische Diagnostik und Therapie bei Herzinfarkt, Colitis ulcerosa und Morbus-Crohn-Patienten. Prax Psychother 3:109–115
Petzold E, Reindell A (1980) Klinische Psychosomatik. Quelle & Mayer, Heidelberg (UTB 991)
Petzold E, Wahl P, Münz R (1985) Was ist gesichert in der Therapie? Diabetes mellitus: Psychosomatik. Arcis, München
Petzold E, Luban-Plozza B, Mattern HJ, Bergmann G (eds) (1987) Brücken von der Psychosomatik zur Allgemeinmedizin. Springer, Berlin Heidelberg New York Tokyo
Pfister O (1921) Vermeintliche Nullen und angebliche Musterkinder. Bircher, Bern
Pflanz M (1962) Sozialer Wandel und Krankheit. Enke, Stuttgart
Platon (o. J.) Charmides. In: Sämtliche Werke, vol 1. Schneider, Berlin
Pöldinger W (1980) Die sogenannte „larvierte Depression“. Ars Medici 5:216–226
Pöldinger W (1982) Differenzieren zwischen Psychosomatosen und larvierten Depressionen. Mk Arzt Fortb 32:53–64
Pöldinger W (1984) Somatisierte Angst und Depressivität. Karger, München Paris London New York Tokyo Sydney
Pöldinger W (1986) Therapie mit Psychopharmaka in der ärztlichen Praxis. Schweiz Ärzteztg 67:2193–2201
Pöldinger W (1987a) Die Sexualität im Alter. MMW 2:3
Pöldinger W (1987b) Behandlung funktioneller sexueller Störungen in der Praxis. MMW 129:35
Pöldinger W, Labhardt F (1988) Sexuell besonders aktiv – denken Sie da an Depression? Sexualmedizin 17:30–34
Pöldinger W, Wider F (1983) Psychopharmakotherapie bei Angstsyndromen, phobischen Syndromen und Zwangssyndromen. In: Langer G, Heimann H (eds) Psychopharmaka. Grundlagen und Therapie. Springer, Berlin Heidelberg New York Tokyo
Pöldinger W, Schmidlin P, Wider F (1983) Index Psychopharmacorum, 6th edn. Huber, Bern Stuttgart Wien
Pöldinger W, Wider F (1986) Die Therapie der Depressionen. Deutscher Ärzte-Verlag, Köln
Prill HJ (1964) Psychosomatische Gynäkologie – Erfahrungen und Ergebnisse einer aktivklinischen Psychotherapie. Urban & Schwarzenberg, München
Pudel V (1976) Verhaltenspsychologische Aspekte der Adipositas. (Referat auf dem Symposium: Diätische, psychologische und soziale Aspekte des Übergewichts. Zürich 8.9. 1976)
Rad M von (1983) Alexithymie – empirische Untersuchungen zur Diagnostik und Therapie psychosomatisch Kranker. Springer, Berlin Heidelberg New York Tokyo
Rad M von, Senf W (1983) Ergebnisforschung in der psychosomatischen Medizin. Urban & Schwarzenberg, München
Radanov B (1983) Problempatienten in der zahnärztlichen Praxis. Schweiz Monatsschr Zahnheilkd 93:812–819
Rallo Romero J, Cabo Casado B de, Olivieri Perdikidis H, Valcarce Avello M (1969) Facteurs psychogènes dans l'arthrose cervicale: syndrome névrotique cervical. Cah Coll Méd Hop Paris 10:205

Reindell A, Petzold E, Kämmerer W, Deter C (1976) Psychotherapie bei Diabetes mellitus? Prax Psychother 21:139–143
Reindell A, Ferner H, Gmelin K (1981) Zur psychosomatischen Differenzierung zwischen Colitis ulcerosa und Ileitis terminalis (Morbus Crohn). Z Psychosom Med Psychoanal 27:358–371
Reisner H (1972) Akute Notfallsituationen in der zahnärztlichen Praxis mit neurologischer und psychiatrischer Symptomatik. Oesterr Z Stomatol 69:318
Richter D, Stauber M (1983) Psychosomatische Probleme in der Geburtshilfe und Gynäkologie. Kehrer, Freiburg
Richter HE, Beckmann D (1969) Herzneurose. Thieme, Stuttgart
Riederer P, Birkmayer W (1980) A new concept: brain area specific imbalance of neurotransmitters in depression syndrome – human brain studies. In: Usdin E, Sourkes TL, Youdim MBH (eds) Enzymes and neurotransmitters in mental disease. Wiley & Sons, New York Chichester
Riemann F (1961) Grundformen der Angst. Reinhaer, Basel München
Rilke RM (1950) The notebook of Malte Lamida Brigge pp 8–9. Translated by John Linton. London, Hogarth Press
Rimon R (1969) A psychosomatic approach to the rheumatoid arthritis. Acta Rheumatol Scand [Suppl 13]
Ringel E (1953) Der Selbstmord: Abschluß einer krankhaften psychischen Entwicklung. Mandrich, Wien Düsseldorf
Ringel E (1969a) Selbstmordverhütung. Huber, Bern Stuttgart Wien
Ringel E (1969b) Klinikerfahrungen in der psychosomatischen Medizin. Wien Klin Wochenschr 81:372–375
Ritschl D, Luban-Plozza B (1987) Die Familie. Risiken und Chancen. Birkhäuser, Basel Boston
Rohracher H (1965) Einführung in die Psychologie, 9th edn. Urban & Schwarzenberg, München Berlin Wien
Rose HK (1976) Die Psychosomatik der Kranken mit normokalzämischer Tetanie. In: Jores A (ed) Praktische Psychosomatik. Huber, Bern Stuttgart Wien, p 256
Rose RM, Jenkins CD, Hurst MW (1978) Health changed in air traffic controllers: a prospective Study. Psychosom Med 40:142–165
Rosenman RH, Friedman M (1959) The possible relationship of the emotions to clinical coronary heart disease. In: Hormones and atherosclerosis. Academic Press, New York
Rubin RT, Mandell AJ (1966) Adrenal cortical activity in pathological emotional states. Am J Psychiatr 123:384–400
Rudolf G (1970) Psychodynamische und psychopathologische Aspekte des Diabetes mellitus. Z Psychosom Med Psychoanal 16:246–262
Sapir M (1975) La formazione psicologica del medico. Etas libri, Milano
Sartre J-P (1945) L'existentialisme est unhumanisme. Nagel, Paris
Satir V (1975) Selbstwert und Kommunikation. Familientherapie für Berater und zur Selbsthilfe. Pfeiffer, München
Schacht J (1974) Zur Psychologie des Hautkranken. Z Klin Psychol Psychother 22:67–85
Schäfer H (1966) Eröffnungsansprache. Verh Dtsch Ges Kreislaufforsch 32:1
Schäfer H (1968) Medizin und Naturwissenschaften. Wehrmed Monatsschr 12:474
Schäfer H (1976) Die Hierarchie der Risikofaktoren. Med Mensch Ges 1:141–146
Schäfer S, Kammerer E, Schröder G (1974) Gruppentherapie zur Reduktion extremer Zahnarztängste bei Kindern. Zahnärztl Prax 25:328, 350b
Schaefer K, Schwarz D (1974) Verhaltenstherapeutische Ansätze für Anorexia nervosa. Z Klin Psychol Psychother 22:267–284
Schärer P (1978) Fallanalyse und Planung: funktionelle Aspekte. Schweiz Monatsschr Zahnheilkd 88:944
Schenker U (1977) Die zahnärztliche Versorgung von Strafgefangenen. Schweiz Monatsschr Zahnheilkd 87:23
Schettler G, Greten H (1978) Koronare Herzkrankheit: Entwicklung in der Bundesrepublik Deutschland und in den USA. Dtsch Ärztebl 75:2263–2266

Schild R (1967) Möglichkeiten und Grenzen psychosomatischer Forschung in der Rheumatologie. Psyche (Stuttg) 38:955
Schild R (1972, 1973a,b) Medizinisch-psychologische Untersuchungen bei Patienten mit rheumatischen Krankheiten, parts I-IV. Psyche (Stuttg) 26:929, 27:50, 27:249
Schlegel L (1963) Allgemeine Betrachtungen zur Psychotherapie in der Allgemeinpraxis. Prax Psychother 8:1
Schmale AH, Iker H (1966) The effect of hopelessness and the development of cancer. Psychosom Med 28:714
Schmidt T (1982) Die Situationshypertonie als Risikofaktor. In: Vaitl D (ed) Essentielle Hypertonie. Springer, Berlin Heidelberg New York
Schneider K (1967) Klinische Psychopathologie, 8th edn. Thieme, Stuttgart
Schüffel W (1978) Auf dem Wege zur patientenbezogenen Medizin. In: Balint E, Luban-Plozza B (eds) Patientenbezogene Medizin. 1. Balint-Methode in der medizinischen Ausbildung. Fischer, Stuttgart New York, p 3
Schüffel W (ed) (1988) Sich gesund fühlen im Jahr 2,000. Der Arzt, sein Patient und die Krankheit, die Technologie, das Team und das System. Springer, Berlin Heidelberg New York Tokyo
Schüffel W, Uexküll T von (1979) Ulcus duodeni. In: Uexküll T von (ed) Lehrbuch der psychosomatischen Medizin. Urban & Schwarzenberg, München Wien Baltimore, p 626
Schulte W (1961) Angstsyndrome. Monatskurse Ärztl Fortbild 11:586
Schultz IH (1970) Das autogene Training, 13th edn. Thieme, Stuttgart
Schultz-Hencke H (1970) Lehrbuch der analytischen Psychotherapie, 2nd edn. Thieme, Stuttgart
Schur M (1974) Zur Metapsychologie der Somatisierung. In: Brede K (ed) Einführung in die psychosomatische Medizin. Fischer Athenäum, Frankfurt am Main, p 335
Schwidder W (1965) Psychosomatik und Psychotherapie bei Störungen und Erkrankungen des Verdauungstraktes. Documenta Geigy, Acta Psychosom 7
Selvini-Palazzoli M (1975) Die Familie des Anorektikers und die Familie des Schizophrenen. Eine transaktionelle Untersuchung. Ehe 107–116
Selvini-Palazzoli M, Boscolo L, Cecchin G, Prata G (1977) Paradoxon und Gegenparadoxon. Klett-Cotta, Stuttgart
Selye H (1946) The general adaption syndrome and the disease of adaption. J Clin Endocrinol 6:117–230
Selye H (1950) The physiology and pathology of exposure to stress. Medical Publications, Montreal
Selye H (1975) Streßbewältigung and Lebensgewinn. Piper, München Zürich
Senarclens M de (1966, 1968) Psyché et pelvis. Gynaecologia (Basel) 28
Senn H (1977) Wahrhaftigkeit am Krankenbett. Schweiz Ärzteztg 7:234–241
Siebeck R (1949) Medizin in Bewegung. Thieme, Stuttgart
Sifneos PE (1973) Problems of psychotherapy of patients with alexithymic characteristics and physical disease. Psychother Psychosom 26:65–70
Slade PD, Russel GFM (1973) Experimental investigations of bodily perception in anorexia nervosa and obesity. Psychother Psychosom 22:359–363
Spitz R (1945, 1946) Hospitalism. Psychoanal Study Child 1:53, 2:68
Spitz RA (1967) Vom Säugling zum Kleinkind. Klett, Stuttgart
Staehelin B (1963) Über die diagnostischen und psychotherapeutischen Möglichkeiten des einfachen Sprechstundengesprächs, dargestellt an drei Fallbeispielen mit Symptomen des Verdauungstraktes. Praxis 52:767–775
Staehelin B (1969) Haben und Sein. Edito academica, Zürich
Stekel W (1920) Die Impotenz des Mannes. Urban & Schwarzenberg, Berlin
Stekel W (1927) Die Geschlechtskälte der Frau, 3rd edn. Urban & Schwarzenberg, Berlin Wien
Stephanos S (1979) Das Konzept des „pensée opératoire" und das „psychosomatische Phänomen". In: Uexküll T von (ed) Lehrbuch der psychosomatischen Medizin. Urban & Schwarzenberg, München Wien Baltimore, p 217

Stieber J, Döhring A, Keil U (1982) Häufigkeit, Bekanntheits- und Behandlungsgrad der Hypertonie in einer Groβstadtbevölkerung. MMW 124, 35:747–752
Stierlin H (1978) Delegation und Familie. Suhrkamp, Frankfurt
Strotzka H (1969) Psychotherapeutische Möglichkeiten in der psychosomatischen Medizin. Wien Klin Wochenschr 20:375–377
Stucke W (ed) (1986) Die Arzt-Patienten-Beziehung im Krankenhaus. Patientenbezogene Medizin 9. Gischer, Stuttgart New York
Szondi L (1968) Freiheit und Zwang im Schicksal des Einzelnen. Huber, Bern Stuttgart Wien
Textor MR (1985) Integrative Familientherapie. Springer, Berlin Heidelberg New York Tokyo
Thiele W (1966) Psychovegetative Syndrome. Sandoz Monographie, Basel
Tournier P (1959) Echtes und falsches Schuldgefühl. Herder, Freiburg
Tournier P (1961) Unsere Maske und wir. Herder, Freiburg
Tournier P (1964) Bibel und Medizin. Herder, Freiburg
Trousseau A (1882) Clinical medicine. Philadelphia
Uexküll T von (1963) Grundfragen der psychosomatischen Medizin. Rowohlt, Reinbek bei Hamburg
Uexküll T von (1969) Funktionelle Syndrome in psychosomatischer Sicht. Wien Klin Wochenschr 81:391
Uexküll T von (ed) (1979) Lehrbuch der psychosomatischen Medizin. Urban & Schwarzenbeck, München Wien Baltimore
Uexküll T von (1982) Zur Psychosomatik der essentiellen Hypertonie – Die Situation als Krankheitsfaktor. In: Köhle K (ed) Zur Psychosomatik von Herz-Kreislauf-Erkrankungen. Forum Galenus Mannheim 8, Heidelberg
Uexküll T von (1988) Theorie der Humanmedizin: Grundlagen ärztlichen Denkens und Handelns. Urban & Schwarzenberg, München
Watzlawik P, Beavin JH, Jackson DD (1972) Menschliche Kommunikation. Huber, Bern
Watzlawik P, Weakland JH (eds) (1980) Interaktion. Huber, Bern
Weimann G (1968) Das Hyperventilationssyndrom. Urban & Schwarzenberg, München Berlin Wien
Weinberg LA (1977, 1979) Evaluation of stress in TJM dysfunction-pain syndrome. J Prosthet Dent 38:192; Schweiz Monatsschr Zahnheilkd 89:239
Weiner H (1977) Psychobiology and human disease. Elesvier, New York
Weiner H, Thaler M, Reiser MF, Mirsky IA (1957) Etiology of duodenal ulcer I – Relation of specific psychological characteristics to rate of gastric secretion (serum pepsinogen). Psychosom Med 19:1
Weintraub A (1969) Der Rücken, psychosomatisch gesehen. Psychosom Med 3:111
Weintraub A (1973) Vertebragene Syndrome aus psychosomatischer Sicht. Fortbildungskurse Rheumatol 2:206–219
Weizsäcker V von (1940, [4]1950) Der Gestaltkreis. Theorie der Einheit von wahrnehmen und bewegen. Thieme, Leipzig (also: Suhrkamp Taschenbuch Wissenschaft, Frankfurt am Main 1973)
Weizsäcker V von (1947) Körpergeschehen und Neurose. Enke, Stuttgart
Weizsäcker V von (1949) Psychosomatische Medizin. Verh Dtsch Ges Inn Med 55:13
Weizsäcker V von (1951) Fälle und Probleme. Enke, Stuttgart
Wesiack W (1976) Anmerkungen zum Verständnis und zur Behandlung der funktionellen Syndrome. Therapiewoche 26:989
Wespi HH (1977) Differentialdiagnose des Lichen ruber planus der Mundschleimhaut und der Leukoplakie. Schweiz Monatsschr Zahnheilkd 87:214
Whitaker CA (1973) My philosophy of psychotherapy. J Contemp Psychother 6:49–52
Wiesenhütter E (1965) Medizinische Psychologie für Vorkliniker, 2nd edn. Urban & Schwarzenberg, München Berlin Wien
Willi J (1975) Die Zweierbeziehung. Rowohlt, Reinbeck bei Hamburg

Willi J (1985) Koevolution. Die Kunst gemeinsamen Wachsens. Rowohlt, Reinbek bei Hamburg
Wirsching M (1979) Familientherapie bei psychosomatischen Krankheiten. In: Hahn P (ed) Psychologie des 20. Jahrhunderts, vol IX. Ergebnisse für die Medizin (1). Psychosomatische Medizin. Kindler, Zürich
Wirsching M, Stierlin H (1982) Krankheit und Familie. Klett-Cotta, Stuttgart
Wittkower ED, Lester EP (1963) Hautkrankheiten in psychosomatischer Sicht. Documenta Geigy. Acta Psychosom 6:1–39
Wolff HG, Wolf S (1943) Human gastric function. Oxford Univ Press, New York London
Wulf M (1932) Über einen interessanten oralen Symptomenkomplex und seine Beziehung zur Sucht. Int Z Psychoanal 18:281–302
Wynne LC (1975) Einige Indikationen und Kontraindikationen für exploratorische Familientherapie. In: Boszormenyi-Nagy I, Framo JL (eds) Familientherapie. Therapie und Praxis, Bd 2. Rowohlt, Reinbek bei Hamburg
Zander W (1976) Vortrag auf der Jahrestagung der Deutschen Psychoanalytischen Gesellschaft e V, November 1976
Zappe HA, Mattern JH, Petzold E (eds) (1988) Brücken von der Allgemeinmedizin zur Psychosomatik. Springer, Berlin Heidelberg New York Tokyo
Zarb GA, Carlsson GE (1979) Temporomandibular joint function and dysfunction. Schweiz Monatsschr Zahnheilkd 89:598
Zellweger H, McDonald JS, Abro G (1968) (cited in: Naturw Rdsch 21:123
Zimmermann H (1977) Zahnärztliche Versorgung alter und behinderter Patienten, die nicht mehr disloziert werden können. Schweiz Monatsschr Zahnheilkd 87:53
Ziolko HU (1971) Zur Psychotherapie eines männlichen Jugendlichen mit Anorexia nervosa. Z Klin Psychol Psychother 19:28–33
Ziolko HU (1985) Bulimie. Z Psychosom Med 31:235–246
Zutt J (1948) Psychiatrische Betrachtungen zur Pubertätsmagersucht. Arch Psychiatr 180:767

Subject Index

GPSR Compliance

The European Union's (EU) General Product Safety Regulation (GPSR) is a set of rules that requires consumer products to be safe and our obligations to ensure this.

If you have any concerns about our products, you can contact us on ProductSafety@springernature.com

In case Publisher is established outside the EU, the EU authorized representative is:

Springer Nature Customer Service Center GmbH
Europaplatz 3
69115 Heidelberg, Germany

Batch number: 10844669

Printed by Printforce, the Netherlands